CHILDBEARING
FAMILIES

This by

For many bereaved parents, the care provided by health professionals at birth – from midwives to antenatal teachers – has a crucial effect on their response to a loss or death. This interactive workbook is clearly applied to practice and has been designed to help practitioners deliver effective bereavement care.

Providing care to grieving parents can be demanding, difficult and stressful, with many feeling ill-equipped to provide appropriate help. Equipping the reader with fundamental skills to support childbearing women, partners and families who have experienced childbirth-related bereavement, this book outlines:

- what bereavement is and the ways in which it can be experienced in relation to pregnancy and birth
- sensitive and supportive ways of delivering bad news to childbearing women, partners and families
- models of grieving
- how to identify when a bereaved parent may require additional support from mental health experts
- ongoing support available for bereaved women, their partners and families
- the impact on practitioners and the support they may require
- how to assess and tailor care to accommodate a range of spiritual and religious beliefs about death.

Written by two highly educated and experienced midwifery lecturers, this practical and evidence-based workbook is a valuable resource for all midwives, neonatal nurses and support workers who work with women in the perinatal period.

Caroline Hollins Martin is Professor of Midwifery at the University of Salford, UK.

Eleanor Forrest is Lecturer in Midwifery at Glasgow Caledonian University, UK.

WITHDRAWN

BEREAVEMENT CARE FOR CHILDBEARING WOMEN AND THEIR FAMILIES

AN INTERACTIVE WORKBOOK

Caroline Hollins Martin and Eleanor Forrest

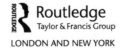

Routledge
Taylor & Francis Group

LONDON AND NEW YORK

First published 2013
by Routledge
2 Park Square, Milton Park, Abingdon, Oxon, OX14 4RN

Simultaneously published in the USA and Canada
by Routledge
711 Third Avenue, New York, NY 10017

Routledge is an imprint of the Taylor & Francis Group, an informa business

British Library Cataloguing in Publication Data
A catalogue record for this book is available from the British Library

Library of Congress Cataloging-in-Publication Data
Hollins Martin, Caroline, author.
Bereavement care for childbearing women and their families : an interactive
workbook/Caroline Hollins Martin and Eleanor Forrest.
p. ; cm.
I. Forrest, Eleanor, author. II. Title.
[DNLM: 1. Stillbirth—psychology—Programmed Instruction. 2.
Bereavement—Programmed Instruction. 3. Caregivers—Programmed
Instruction. 4. Family Relations—Programmed Instruction. 5. Fetal Death—
Programmed Instruction. 6. Women—psychology—Programmed Instruction.
WQ 18.2]
RG648
618.3'9—dc23
2013002743

ISBN13: 978-0-415-82723-2 (hbk)
ISBN13: 978-0-415-82724-9 (pbk)
ISBN13: 978-0-203-36696-7 (ebk)

Typeset in Sabon by
FiSH Books Ltd, Enfield

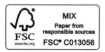

MIX
Paper from
responsible sources
FSC   FSC® C013056
www.fsc.org

Printed and bound in Great Britain by
TJ International Ltd, Padstow, Cornwall

Contents

Acknowledgements

EARTH MOTHER

The painting 'Earth Mother' on the front cover of this book was painted by Becca Marsh who has a BA(Hons) in Fine Art and was a student midwife at the University of Salford. She qualified in September 2012, and is now working at Royal Bolton Hospital as a midwife. The painting was completed as part of the 'The Art of Midwifery' project, which is carried out in the third year of the midwifery degree programme. The art project involves students creating positive images of pregnancy and birth.

SPECIAL THANKS

The authors would like to thank the following people who contributed to the book through discussions and by providing information. These included:

- Cindy Horan, a midwife at Southern General Maternity Hospital and provides a priceless counselling service to the bereaved women of Glasgow;
- Linda Wylie, a lecturer in midwifery at the University of West of Scotland;
- Dr Maria Pollard, a senior lecturer in midwifery at the University of West of Scotland;
- Elma Paxton, a former midwifery lecturer at Glasgow Caledonian University;
- Dr Ewan Kelly, a part-time senior lecturer and programme director for healthcare chaplaincy and spiritual care at NHS Education for Scotland (NES);
- all the student midwives at the University of Salford, Glasgow Caledonian University and the University of West of Scotland, who were participants in the pilot evaluation of the initial workbook.

The authors

Caroline J. Hollins Martin PhD MPhil BSc ADM PGCE RMT RM RGN MBPsS is a Professor in Midwifery in the College of Health and Social Care at the University of Salford. Her background has encompassed a career in women's reproductive health that spans 26 years. The first 11 of these were spent as a clinical midwife in Ayrshire (Scotland) and the remaining 15 were spent teaching and researching women's reproductive health within universities. She is an NMC-registered midwife and

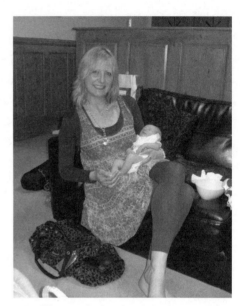

Caroline with Jamie Ralston McKay Welsh

lecturer/practice educator. She is also a graduate and postgraduate in psychology and a Member of the British Psychological Society (MBPsS). Her research interests lie in social psychology that relates to women's reproductive health, with much of her work relating to obstructing autonomy, evidenced-based practice and providing choice and control to childbearing women. More recently, focus has shifted to developing useful tools for maternal health practitioners to use in clinical practice; for example, the Birth Participation Scale (BPS) to assess fathers fears and needs in relation to childbirth and the Birth Satisfaction Scale (BSS) to assess mothers' perceptions of their birth experience. Current research interests lie in shaping perinatal bereavement care, outcomes of maternal activity during labour and the effects of music upon women's stress levels. To date, she has published 40 peer-reviewed papers, presented 36 conference papers, written four book chapters and is an associate editor for women's reproductive health papers submitted to the *Journal of Nurse Education in Practice*.

Dedication

I would like to dedicate this book to Willow, my own maternal bereavement (shared with Colin Martin), my mother Margaret Hollins who died in tragic circumstances and my father, the late Reverend Roger Hollins; all of whom are in spirit. I would also like to thank Arnold Burgoyne for his help and support.

Eleanor Forrest MPhil BScN ECHN PGCE RMT RM was born and brought up in Scotland and trained as a nurse and midwife in Glasgow. Over the last 27 years she has lived and worked in a variety of countries and midwifery environments. Her Master of Philosophy was about women's experiences and perceptions of service 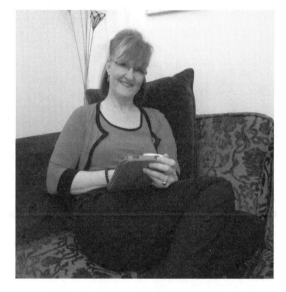 provision for women who are experiencing postnatal depression. Much of her clinical experience as a midwife has focused on providing holistic care to women with mental health problems and their families during the perinatal period. Eleanor was the first midwife to provide a specialist service that provides for childbearing women with perinatal mental health problems in Glasgow. Through working with women in this capacity she has recognised that adaptation to motherhood often involves a process of grieving, even when a healthy infant has been born.

Currently, Eleanor works as a lecturer in midwifery at Glasgow Caledonian University. She is involved in delivering modules she has written for multi-professional perinatal mental health practitioners. She also lectures on the undergraduate midwifery programme and delivers international postgraduate Master's modules using a virtual learning environment. Eleanor has also contributed to the book *Becoming a Midwife* by adding a discussion about midwives and perinatal mental health.

Dedication
My life's journey would not be so colourful without my wonderful children Sean and Olivia who taught me everything about being a mother. I dedicate this book to them.

Foreword

Midwifery, like all of medicine, moves rapidly forward with technical progress and reorganisation of systems. In this process the patient and relatives can easily be forgotten. This will not happen if you read this book, and certainly not for bereavement care in midwifery.

Giving patients or relatives bad news, especially about the loss of a life, is never easy, not for those receiving it nor for those giving it. The kind word, the reassurance, the understanding, the explanation and the holding of the hand – the values we were brought up with – remain just as essential as ever. But now we need even more.

Some of us are good at passing on bad news and some are not. I always found it difficult, and I, like many, developed my skills from learning through experience, unfortunately making mistakes on the way. How much better to learn from the experience of others? You can do that from reading this book.

This book is more than a workbook; it is an excellent analysis and explanation of all that is involved in the care of bereaved women and their families. It deals with a variety of subjects such as grief, cultural diversity and imparting bad news. I hope it is read not only by midwives but by many others involved in the care of patients and their relatives.

Sam Galbraith

Sam Galbraith was a consultant neurosurgeon at the Institute of Neurological Sciences in Glasgow until 1988, when he was elected as Member of Parliament for Strathkelvin and Bearsden. Following the 1997 general election he was Parliamentary Under-Secretary of State at the Scottish Office, where he was Minister for Health, Sport and the Arts. Subsequently, he was elected to the first Scottish Parliament in 1999. He retired from Westminster and Holyrood in 2001.

Preface

Maternity health and social care professionals are often called upon to care for parents who have experienced a pregnancy loss or the death of an infant. In such circumstances they are expected to interact with bereaved parents and their families in a supportive manner. Consequently, it is important that staff feel adequately prepared with strategies to deliver effective bereavement care.

The Stillbirth and Neonatal Death Society (SANDS) recommends that all community health practitioners who support bereaved parents should have access to basic, post-basic and in-service training to equip them to offer adequate care to such families (SANDS, 2009). This has recently been endorsed by the Scottish government's guidance 'Shaping Bereavement Care' (2011), which called for improved training and support for all NHS staff working in this field. For many bereaved parents, the care that maternity health and social care professionals provide has a crucial effect on their response to a loss or death (Engler and Lasker, 2000; Rowa-Dewar, 2002). Providing care to grieving parents can be demanding, difficult and stressful (Gensch and Midland, 2000; Säflund *et al.*, 2004), with some professionals feeling ill-equipped to provide appropriate help (Robinson *et al.*, 1999). In 2009, the National Maternity Support Foundation (NMSF) survey reported that the level of bereavement care delivered in a number of maternity units in the UK was inadequate:

> It is clear that there is a somewhat 'patchy' approach to bereavement midwife care with an apparent lack of national strategy and clear up-to-date guidelines.
>
> (NMSF, 2009: 12)

In response to the results of the NMSF (2009), two experienced midwifery lecturers from two universities (University of Salford and Glasgow Caledonian University) collaborated to write this book. This workbook has been designed to facilitate midwives, neonatal nurses and allied health and social care professionals in developing structured skills to deliver effective bereavement care. On completion of this workbook the reader should be equipped with fundamental skills to support childbearing women, partners and families who have experienced childbirth-related bereavement. Contents were specifically designed to educate maternity healthcare providers at undergraduate level in the UK. However, the subject matter may prove useful for updating/coaching/tutoring a variety of allied health and social care providers. At a universal and international level, there is valuable information for a wide range of interested parties.

Introduction

Grief is a multifaceted response to the loss of someone or something to which a bond has been formed. Although conventionally focused on the emotional response to loss, it also has physical, cognitive, behavioural, social, spiritual and philosophical dimensions. While terms are often used interchangeably, 'bereavement' refers to the state of loss, and 'grief' to the reaction to the loss of someone or something important. For example, someone important could mean a miscarriage or stillbirth and something important could be the social identity of potential motherhood lost when a baby is adopted. The term bereavement encompasses grief and mourning and denotes the emotions and behaviour of a childbearing woman who has suffered a loss. A childbearing woman who has experienced a loss may be said to go through a bereavement period, which is the time it takes to grieve and adjust to the loss. Every bereavement process is specific to each childbearing woman, partner and family dependent upon their attachment and beliefs surrounding their loss. Grief expressed signals the emotional responses invoked by the loss. Mourning refers to actions customarily associated with grief, such as styles of crying and lamenting the loss. Childbearing women and their families who have experienced a loss in varying degrees will experience grief. As such, maternity care professionals should be familiar with the various ways of supporting women and families when they are experiencing bereavement. Midwives and neonatal nurses do not care for bereaved parents in isolation; they are part of a collaborative team that may include doctors, chaplains, bereavement officers and counsellors, registrars, funeral directors, representatives of faith communities, voluntary support agencies and, of course, family and friends.

Pregnancy loss is a form of 'disenfranchised grief' (Bartellas and Van Aerde, 2003), with many parents recognising that sometimes it is not socially acceptable to talk about the miscarriage or stillbirth they have experienced. As a consequence, they may feel isolated from and misunderstood by friends, family and colleagues (Kelly, 2007). The impact of loss and bereavement on an individual's spiritual wellbeing can be profound. A person's sense of meaning and understanding of the world can be called into question. Existential questions such as 'Why?, Why me?', 'Why now?', 'What have I done to deserve this?' or 'If there is a God, how can God allow this to happen?' are commonly expressed (Kelly, 2007). The bereaved are not looking for answers to these questions, but often appreciate time and space provided by a non-judgemental other to express and explore these issues. Other symptoms of spiritual distress are a sense of hopelessness, helplessness, lack of control, and struggles with identity, purpose and role. Questions may be asked like, 'If I am no longer a wife, mother or son, then who am I?'

For most who experience bereavement, no professional support is required, whilst others may decide to seek supplementary support from appropriately trained professionals. Grief counselling, professional support groups, educational classes and peer-led support groups are resources available to the bereaved. Where grief has occurred in consequence to a childbearing event, the midwife is usually the first point of contact. It is therefore important that all maternity care professionals are equipped with appropriate knowledge about how best to support a woman, her partner and her family in this position.

Crying is a normal and natural part of grieving, as is talking about the loss experience. If forced or excessive, grief can become harmful. George Bonanno conducted a research study that focused on grief and trauma (Bonanno, 2009). Bonanno's subjects experienced loss through war, terrorism, death of a child, premature death of a spouse, sexual abuse, childhood diagnoses of AIDS, and other devastating loss and trauma events. He found that people have an innate resilience in the event of grief and trauma events.

Kübler-Ross (1969, 2005) developed a theory that incorporates five discrete stages by which people deal with loss. These are denial, anger, bargaining, depression and acceptance (Figure I.1). The theory purports that the stages comprise a framework that facilitates people to learn to live without what they have lost. Midwives may use the Kübler-Ross model or a similar framework to help them identify and understand what a childbearing woman who has suffered a loss may be feeling. The incorporated stages are not discrete entities on a linear timeline of grief, and not every bereaved childbearing woman will progress through all five stages in the prescribed sequence. The Kübler-Ross five-stage model of

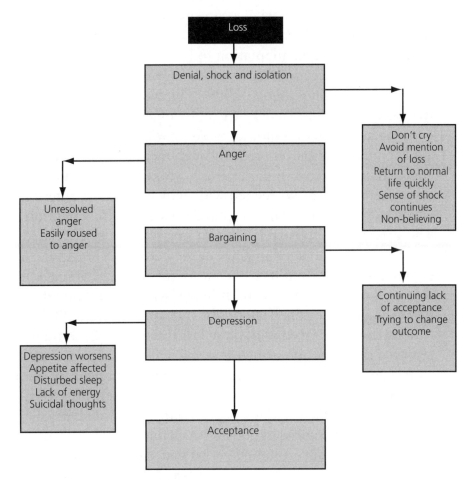

Figure I.1 Grief stages

grieving has been credited with bringing mainstream awareness to the sensitivities required for better treatment of people who are dealing with loss. More recently, researchers have developed several new models or theories to help professionals understand the processes of bereavement. These models serve to facilitate professionals who are involved in supporting the bereaved by providing a knowledge base from which to practise. For example, Worden's (1983) tasks of bereavement provide a framework to guide grief work, while the dual process model demonstrates the need to deal with both the primary loss and secondary stressors (Stroebe and Schut, 1999). No model of grieving is recommended above another, as all have mechanisms that may be helpful towards aiding understanding of the bereavement process and the processes involved in adaptation to loss.

A physical reaction to bereavement precedes any psychological symptoms (O'Connor et al., 2009). Functional Magnetic Resonance Imaging (FMRI) scans of women who have experienced death of a mother or sister within five years identified a local inflammation response through measuring salivary concentrations of pro-inflammatory cytokines. Production of these chemicals was correlated with activation in the anterior cingulate cortex and orbitofrontal cortex of the human brain. This activation also correlated with free recall of grief-related word stimuli; that is, talking about the bereavement experience stimulates feelings and its associated expression. This suggests that grief can cause stress and is linked with the emotional processing parts of the frontal lobe (O'Connor et al., 2009). Among those bereaved within the last three months, those who reported thoughts about their loss showed ventral amygdala and rostral anterior cingulate cortex hyperactivity. In the case of the amygdala, this links to sadness intensity. In those who avoid thoughts about their loss, there is a related opposite type of pattern in neurological responses (O'Connor et al., 2009).

The rationale underpinning why a maternity care professional should complete this workbook is because their role encompasses responsibility for delivering holistic evidence-based care to childbearing women. Consequently, it is important to recognise the physical, psychological and social components of bereavement, loss and grief and to be equipped with appropriate skills to handle related adversity.

PURPOSE OF THIS INTERACTIVE WORKBOOK

This workbook will be a valuable resource for all maternity care providers, especially those who provide bereavement support to childbearing women, and for lecturers who educate student professionals for their future role as clinicians. The content of this workbook represents the highest quality of care provision that is prescribed in western cultures. Essentially, what is encompassed is underpinned by evidenced-based protocols of the United Kingdom. As such, it must be recognised that some of the prescribed pathways of care may not be suitable for delivery according to the social, religious and cultural systems of all communities in the world. Threaded throughout the workbook, an emphasis is placed upon the importance of providing individualised care to meet the particularised needs of the person at the centre of the loss. As such, importance is placed on providing choice and control to the experiencer of grief. This does not devalue the worth of this workbook, which represents the highest offerable standard of bereavement care, which may not, in fact, be economically viable to deliver in all maternity units of the UK or less economically privileged countries. Nonetheless, the international reader may find it enlightening to embrace how an alternative society manages perinatal bereavement care. Besides, when writing educational curriculum, the majority of writers of programmes embrace cross-cultural studies. *Per se*, this widens readership of this workbook to an international level. To view the learning objectives (LO) encompassed within this workbook, see Table I.1.

Table I.1 Learning objectives (LO) to shape bereavement care of maternity care providers and allied health and social care providers in practice

(LO1) Classify areas of maternity care that incur bereavement.

(LO2) Discuss sensitive and supportive processes of delivering bad news to childbearing women, partners and families.

(LO3) Critically appraise the procedures categorised on a bereavement protocol.

(LO4) Critically appraise the models of grieving.

(LO5) Recognise instances where a childbearing woman's grief process has become dysfunctional and help is required from mental health experts.

(LO6) Outline processes involved in caring for and advising a bereaved woman/partner/family about how to access ongoing support on discharge from maternity care.

(LO7) Recognise where a bereavement incident may affect a member of staff adversely.

(LO8) Assess individual women/partner/family's spiritual/religious beliefs and adapt bereavement care to accommodate.

1

Areas of maternity care that incur bereavement

Learning objective addressed

On completion of Chapter 1 the reader should be able to:

1. Classify areas of maternity care that incur bereavement.

1.1 AREAS OF MATERNITY CARE THAT INCUR BEREAVEMENT

The death of a child can take the form of a loss in pregnancy, the perinatal period or infancy. For example:

- early pregnancy loss such as ectopic pregnancy and miscarriage
- stillbirth
- perinatal death
- neonatal death
- sudden infant death syndrome (SIDS)
- death of an older child.
- infertility.

In the majority of cases, parents experience acute grief. The death of a child could be considered to be one of the most intense forms of grief and one of the hardest to bear (Shane, 1992). For the majority, the death of a child is an event that evokes unbearable anguish and sorrow (Stack, 2003). A childbearing woman does not simply get over her loss; instead, she will need to adapt and learn to live with it. Interventions and support can make all the difference to the fortitude of a parent in this type of grief, with risk factors such as family break-up or suicide a potential outcome. Feelings of responsibility, whether legitimate or not, are omnipresent. Also, the nature of the parent–infant relationship may result in an assortment of problems, as women, partners and families seek to cope with their loss. Parents who suffer miscarriage or a regretful termination of pregnancy may experience resentment towards others who have accomplished successful pregnancies.

OTHER LOSSES
Parents may grieve due to loss experienced through events other than death. For example:

■ having a child adopted or fostered
■ termination of a pregnancy for medical or social reasons
■ loss of a healthy child through prematurity, illness or abnormality
■ legal termination of parental rights incited by the social work department
■ having a history of child abuse, neglect or incompetent parenting
■ loss of paternal identity due to separation from the childbearing woman
■ loss of a romantic relationship (i.e. divorce or break-up)
■ for a childbearing woman who strongly identifies with her occupation, a sense of grief from having to discontinue or alter work arrangements due to parenting responsibilities
■ a loss of trust, which may also constitute a form of grief.

Each society has its own particular cultural approaches to managing bereavement within the community. These include specific rituals, styles of dress and habits, as well as attitudes that the bereaved are expected to follow. For example, in China where Buddhism guides the majority of citizens, devotees continue their ties with the deceased through religious rituals that express continued attachment. Some of these customs involve presenting plates of conscientiously prepared food and bestowing gifts of cardboard replicas of essential domestic items for use in the spirit world; for example, clothes, shoes, cars, houses and bags of paper money. The significant other proceeds to burn these cardboard items in an incinerator provided by the monks who dwell within the Buddhist temple. The underpinning belief is that the deceased loved one will bestow good fortune upon the initiator and guide them towards positive action here in the physical world. In contrast, amongst the Hopi people of Arizona, the deceased are swiftly forgotten and life continues. In essence, different cultures grieve in different ways and these will be discussed in more detail in Chapter 7. Also, later on in this workbook you will be looking at some of the rituals that maternity care professionals in the UK undertake when dealing with loss of a baby in clinical practice.

1.2 WHAT IS A STILLBIRTH?

Stillbirth is the label given to a fetus who has died *in utero*. A stillborn is a baby who is born dead after 24 completed weeks of pregnancy. If the baby dies before 24 completed weeks, it is known as a *late miscarriage*. Stillbirths are not uncommon, with approximately 4,000 occurring every year in the UK.

- 1 in 200 births in the UK conclude in stillbirth.
- 11 babies born in the UK are stillborn every day.
- In the UK, stillbirth occurs ten times more often than cot death.

The majority of *stillbirths* arise in full-term pregnancies.

WHAT ARE THE CAUSES OF STILLBIRTH?

A post mortem does not always elicit cause of death, with 50 per cent of stillbirths remaining undiagnosed. Possible instigators of stillbirth include:

- maternal health problems, e.g. intrahepatic cholestasis, diabetes, hypertension, pre-eclampsia, eclampsia etc.
- maternal drug addiction

- anoxia due to placenta or umbilical cord malfunction, e.g. placental abruption, placenta praevia, true knot in cord, cord prolapse, short cord (<30 cm), long cord (>70 cm), cord entanglement
- rhesus disease
- bacterial infection
- congenital defects, e.g. pulmonary hypoplasia
- congenital abnormality
- intra uterine growth retardation (IUGR)
- trauma, e.g. road traffic accidents (RTA)
- radiation exposure
- twin competition for intrauterine resources or cord entanglement.

The concept of carrying a deceased fetus may be traumatic for the woman, with immediate induction being the solution. The mother is usually expected to labour and give birth vaginally, quite simply because caesarian section increases risk of complications and produces a uterine scar that may in future rupture. A caesarian birth is only recommended when vaginal birth is predicted to be or has become problematic. A pregnancy may be purposely terminated late when the fetus has been diagnosed with a congenital abnormality that is incompatible with life. In such circumstances UK law expects the infant to be registered as a stillbirth.

DIAGNOSIS OF STILLBIRTH
It is usual for fetal activity to be consistent, with alterations in the number and style of movements signposting fetal distress. Kick charts can be used to detect changes in fetal activity, with cardiotocography (CTG) and ultrasound used to clinch a diagnosis of fetal death.

PREVENTING STILLBIRTH
Quality preconception and antenatal care can work towards reducing disease through early detection and treatment of

complications. But with this approach many causes of stillbirth remain unknown, which makes deterrence an arduous task. Nevertheless, there are some strategies that maternity experts can implement to reduce the risk of stillbirth. These include promptly treating maternal:

- infection
- hypertension
- diabetes
- drug use.

In addition, quality health education plays a part. Ordinarily, a stillbirth does not present health risks to the childbearing woman, with labour usually initiating itself two weeks post-death. After this time period, labour must be induced to remove the threat of maternal blood clotting.

1.3 DEFINING THE TERMS 'FETAL MORTALITY', 'NEONATAL MORTALITY', 'INFANT MORTALITY RATE' AND 'PERINATAL MORTALITY RATE'

(A) FETAL MORTALITY
Fetal mortality encompasses any death of a fetus after 20 weeks' gestation or above 500 grams in weight. Fetal death is also usually divided into death prior to labour *(antepartum death)* and death during labour *(intrapartum death)*.

(B) NEONATAL MORTALITY
(i) *Early neonatal mortality* refers to a death of a live-born baby within the first seven days of life.
(ii) *Late neonatal mortality* refers to a death of a live-born baby after seven days until before 28 days.
Neonatal mortality is the sum of the above (i) and (ii).

(C) INFANT MORTALITY RATE
Neonatal mortality and *postneonatal mortality* (which covers the

remaining 11 months of the first year of life) are reflected in the *infant mortality rate*.

(D) PERINATAL MORTALITY RATE

The perinatal mortality rate refers to the number of perinatal deaths per 1,000 total births. It is usually reported on an annual basis. It is a key marker used to measure the effectiveness of healthcare delivery. Comparing differing perinatal mortality rates is hindered by changeable definitions, registration bias and differences in underpinning risks between populations, cultures and nations. Perinatal mortality rates vary widely and are below ten per 1,000 total births in some developed countries and more than ten times higher in some developing countries.

1.4 DEFINING THE TERMS 'LOSS', 'GRIEF' AND 'BEREAVEMENT'

Consider what the following terms mean to you:

- loss
- grief
- bereavement.

Activity 1

Consider what the terms 'loss', 'grief' and 'bereavement' mean to you.

Loss..

....

....

Grief..

....

....

Bereavement ....

....

....

Now let us consider formal definitions of loss, grief and bereavement and how midwives can better understand the feelings experienced by childbearing women, their partners and family members.

WHAT IS LOSS?

Loss is defined as the severing or breaking of an attachment to someone or something that results in a changed relationship. Two general categories of loss exist: 1. physical loss, and 2. psychological loss. A physical loss is the loss of something tangible. For example:

- a car that is stolen
- a house that burns down
- a precious belonging that has been mislaid.

One might assume that the possessor may have emotions in response to that loss. In contrast, a psychological loss is a symbolic loss and features something intangible and psychosocial in nature. For example:

- experiencing a divorce
- retiring
- developing an unremitting illness
- having one's fantasy or dream wiped out.

WHAT IS PERINATAL LOSS?

The legal definition of perinatal loss is a stillbirth beyond 24 weeks' gestation or death of an infant in the first week of life. In response to such an event it is common for the mother to experience emotions such as fear, anxiety and helplessness, which requires sensitive handling and appropriate discussion with the midwife (Shane, 1992). During such an event, the care that maternity care professionals provide may have a crucial effect on the parent's response to their loss (Engler and Lasker, 2000). Caring for and supporting parents who have lost a baby can be extremely demanding, difficult and stressful (Billson and Tyrrell, 2003).

Much of the published literature includes references to perinatal loss and bereavement care in western societies (Caelli *et al.*, 2002; Engler *et al.*, 2004; Engler and Lasker, 2000; Gardner, 1999; Gensch and Midland, 2000; Lin and Lasker, 1996; Shane, 1992). Most of this research has focused on parental grief responses and interventions that facilitate parental adaptation to their loss (Blackburn and Copley, 1989; Brost and Kenney, 1992).

Just as no two deaths are alike, so it is with grief and bereavement. To the childbearing woman, partner, family and friends, bereavement causes great stress that can temporarily impair concentration, decision-making and performance. Without adequate support, grief and bereavement may affect a person's health. But with sufficient support, the experience of grief and bereavement can enhance an individual's personal growth and facilitate development of their understanding about the meaning of life.

However, as has been mentioned, perinatal loss does not only relate to a death. You may not consider that some events within midwifery practice are potential provoker's of grief. Examples may include:

- loss of a normal labour due to the childbearing woman requiring an emergency caesarean section
- loss of a healthy, normal-sized baby when the infant has been born extremely premature
- loss of one's uterus due to essential removal to alleviate postpartum haemorrhage.

WHAT IS GRIEF?

Grief refers to the process of experiencing psychological, behavioural, social and physical reactions to the perception of loss. Five important clinical implications derive from this definition:

Activity 2

(a) Identify a loss that you have experienced and classify your reactions in terms of psychological, behavioural, social and physical responses:

Psychological responses to grief..

....

....

Behavioural responses to grief ....

....

....

Social responses to grief ....

....

....

Physical responses to grief ....

....

....

Spiritual responses to grief..

....

....

(b) Identify a loss that a childbearing woman has experienced and classify her reactions in terms of psychological, behavioural, social and physical. If you have not encountered a situation akin to this, read around the topic. Such responses are discussed later in this workbook.

Psychological responses to grief..

....

....

Behavioural responses to grief ....

....

....

Social responses to grief ....

....

....

Physical responses to grief ....

....

....

Spiritual responses to grief ....

....

....

1. Grief is experienced in five major ways:
   - psychologically
   - behaviourally
   - socially
   - physically
   - spiritually.
2. Grief is a systematic process that involves several emotional states. It is not motionless and stationary. In other words, it actively incorporates change over time.
3. Grief is a normal expectable response to a loss. The absence of it could in some situations be considered abnormal or even pathological.
4. Grief is a reaction to all types of loss. It is not just about fatality. Death of a baby in midwifery practice is only one example of loss.
5. Grief is dependent upon the childbearing woman's unique perception of her loss. It is not necessary for this loss to be socially recognised or validated by others for her to grieve. It is, however, helpful for midwives to recognise the possibility that it may happen.

A childbearing woman's response to a significant loss will usually express one or all of the following five dimensions:

1. her feelings about the loss, e.g. sadness, despair, remorse
2. her objection to the loss and wish to reverse the situation, e.g. anger, searching, fixation with what has happened
3. the effects on her as a direct result of the loss, e.g. disorganisation, bewilderment, horror, anxiety state and/or physical symptoms (loss of appetite, palpitations, nausea etc.)
4. her response behaviours to the loss, e.g. crying, social withdrawal, use of medication, drugs and/or alcohol
5. existential questions about the loss may be asked; for example, wrestling with 'why' the loss might have happened. A search for 'why' questions may call into question the way the bereaved understood the world prior to their loss.

Grief is a natural response to loss and it incorporates a range of reactions. Associated emotions include:

- sadness
- anger
- guilt
- pain
- longing for the lost person or thing.

A grief reaction may be experienced following:

- the end of a relationship
- moving away from home
- loss of a fantasy or dream.

Grief is painful to experience and witness, with the majority of people innately equipped to adapt and survive their loss.

Grieving is about coming to terms with a loss. The length of time it takes for an individual to adjust is variable. Adaptation can depend on several factors:

- the significance of the loss to the person concerned
- the character of the loss
- other events running simultaneously to the loss
- prior experience of loss.

Although there may be similarities in people's responses, there can also be marked differences. Each person grieves and recovers in their personal way.

WHAT IS BEREAVEMENT?

Bereavement is the total reaction to a loss and includes the process of healing and recovery from the loss. Bereavement results in a great longing for the lost person or object and requires a period of adjustment by the experiencer that may take years. All parts of the bereaved individual may be affected. This includes emotional, physical, spiritual and social aspects of that person. The overriding feeling is ordinarily one of intense pain, which is otherwise known as grief.

Activity 3

Consider your own situation or someone you know and how they responded to a significant loss.

The loss event ....

1. Associated feelings about the loss, e.g. sadness, despair, remorse .....
....
....

2. Objections to the loss and wish to reverse the situation, e.g. anger, searching, fixation with what has happened ....
....
....
....

3. Effects that directly resulted from the loss, e.g. disorganisation, bewilderment, horror, anxiety state and/or physical symptoms (loss of appetite, palpitations, nausea etc.) ....
....
....
....

4. Individual response behaviours, e.g. crying, social withdrawal, use of medication/drugs/alcohol ....
....
....
....

5. Existentialist questions asked? ....
....
....
....

Activity 4

Identify a loss that caused you grief ....

....

What strategies did you use to help you cope?

....

....

....

....

....

Which of these strategies were beneficial?

....

....

....

Which of these strategies were detrimental?

....

....

....

CONCLUSION

The objective of this chapter is to examine areas of maternity care provision that incur bereavement for the purpose of laying down foundation slabs for related discourse in subsequent chapters. Having a stillborn baby or perinatal death is an experience that is unimaginably painful for parents. Grief for the baby can take a number of forms. The couple should be provided with opportunities for counselling, which they may find a great source of help. Health and social care professionals can help with subsequent grieving by exampling to parents and family how to put together a:

- special memory pack
- book of dedication to the lost infant containing stories, poems and pictures
- memorial garden

■ remembrance service for important dates like birthdays.

The mother is always asked to provide permission for a post mortem to be conducted on her stillborn baby. This can be a traumatic decision, with some wishing to know exactly why their infant died and others wanting their infant to be left intact. Registration of the birth and/or death, and having a funeral, is a legal requirement for all stillborn babies, even when the parents elect not to attend these events. Maternity units have specialist bereavement services to advise, assist and support parents with decision-making during this difficult time. Registering the birth will provide parents with the opportunity to acknowledge their infant's existence and is also essential for statistical records and research. Stillbirths must be registered at the maternity unit or at the local registry office within 42 days of death and not more than three months post-event.

It is understandably demanding to know how best to support and show sympathy to the childbearing woman, partner and family experiencing the loss, especially when so many couples in your care have had successful pregnancies and outcomes. Main aspects to advise relatives and friends about include:

■ not avoiding contact, as bereaved parents can become isolated
■ acknowledging the infant's death in person, by telephone, sending a card, email and/or text at repeated intervals
■ always referring to the baby by its given name
■ listening when the bereaved person wants to talk.

Take cues from the couple, with some desiring to be surrounded by familiar people and others finding it difficult to be around healthy pregnant women and newborn babies. There are a myriad of psychological processes surrounding perinatal bereavement addressed in this workbook. The first steps discussed in Chapter 2 involve the perceptive and compassionate processes involved in imparting the shocking information of a problem or death to the childbearing woman, partner and family.

2

Breaking bad news

Learning objective addressed

On completion of Chapter 2 the reader should be able to:

2. Discuss sensitive and supportive processes of delivering bad news to childbearing women, partners and families.

2.1 BREAKING BAD NEWS

Breaking bad news to women and their families is an inevitable part of a maternity care professional's role, especially when working with those who are experiencing a difficult pregnancy or loss. As such, it is imperative that providers of care are aware of the importance of being a good communicator, and that they know how to impart difficult information in a sensitive manner. Cases that involve breaking bad news include fetal compromise, or demise, and the woman, her partner and her family may be unaware, or fully aware, of the situation and its implications. In such situations, it is the professional's duty to impart salient information and provide referral and support networks to those involved. In doing so, a fine balance is required between causing pain and distress and providing essential knowledge. A sensitive and informative approach will initiate processes for those involved coming to terms with their loss.

When problems arise, childbearing women are often transferred to a hospital that has specialised neonatal facilities, where best possible care can be provided to the childbearing woman, partner and baby. Although the woman may be aware of complications, she may not have full cognition of the extent of the problem and its potential outcomes. Misinterpretations and misconstructions can make this a perplexing time for those at the centre of care provision. Once investigations have taken place to update and confirm the impediments involved, the midwife may be considered the right person to break the bad news to the family. It is imperative that midwives are prepared for such events and that they plan an appropriate time and venue to impart information to the childbearing woman, partner and family. For example, a side room with attractive and comfortable chairs, bathroom facilities, away from the sounds of mothers with healthy crying babies and external telephone calls. Upon receiving difficult and perhaps complex details, the couple must be afforded time to absorb information in a safe environment. Such action will facilitate healthy commencement of the grieving process.

The woman may have been referred from home or an outlying clinic for ultrasound to confirm the suspected diagnosis. In order to be fully prepared for such events, the maternity care provider should ensure that relevant background information is available; for example, a midwife or general practitioner referral letter and the childbearing woman's case records. Schedule in an appointed amount of time to ensure that appropriate attention is paid to the woman's needs. An unfitting time would be in the middle of a busy clinic, where there are countless interruptions and distractions. Providing accommodation for a supportive significant other is paramount to the troubled and grieving woman's companionship needs. If the deliverer is prepared in advance about the type of bad news to be broken, they can decide whether another type of allied professional is required to provide additional information – for example, a specialist midwife, social worker, nurse or doctor. If the woman is oblivious to the gravity of the situation, she may have elected to attend the maternity unit unaccompanied. In this instance, it may be relevant to contact an individual of her choice to provide more intimate support.

Before breaking bad news, the deliverer must elucidate on the childbearing woman's precise understandings of her situation.

This may be achieved through the use of the following probing, open-ended questions:

1. What have you been told so far?
2. What has happened since your last appointment?
3. How have things been for you?

Listening is a skill that the deliverer must use during the communication event. At all times the childbearing woman must be at the centre of the communication. The communicator must not trivialise the communication event with irrelevant conversation about mundane, inconsequential events that do not relate to the issue in hand. This is particularly relevant when breaking bad news, with displays of empathy crucial to developing trust and showing that staff care. Figure 2.1 depicts an empathetic cycle of listening.

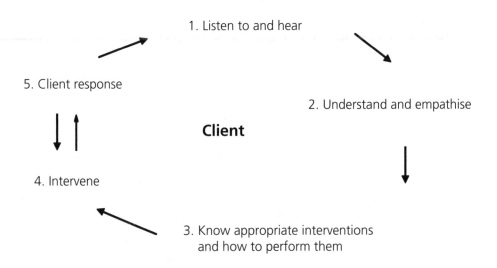

Figure 2.1 Empathetic cycle of listening

The information given at the 'breaking bad news' event is a snapshot that is likely to be replayed repeatedly in the childbearing woman's mind. This makes the communication event momentous, with irrevocable implications. In light of this possibility, it is essential that the deliverer is professional, supportive and demonstrates sincere and genuine empathy.

It is recommended that a fairly direct approach be taken when breaking bad news. The couple may have intuitively recognised that something is amiss and therefore one must not prevaricate and protract anguish. ARC (2012) proposes some example statements that will indicate the serious nature of the situation:

1. I do have something to tell you.
2. I am afraid it is more serious than we expected.
3. I am very sorry to have to tell you.
4. It is not very good news I am afraid.

Once bad news has been given, there is a range of potential emotional and behavioural responses that may be displayed between re-assimilation and regularity being resumed. The emotional process during the breaking bad news event is the beginning of the grief process, which is customarily exhibited in different phases (see Chapter 3). More often the initial response is: 1. shock, which may incorporate feelings of numbness, denial, disbelief, hysteria and inability to think cohesively; 2. protest, whereby an individual may have strong, powerful feelings of anger, guilt, sadness, fear, yearning and searching for answers; and, as the reality and enormity of the situation is acknowledged; 3. disorganisation of emotions. During this phase, the woman may experience feelings of overwhelming bleakness, despair, apathy, anxiety and confusion. Having passed through the three preceding stages of: shock, protest and dis-organisation, once re-organisation of the facts have begun to be assimilated, there is a gradual return to more ordinary functioning. To view a diagrammatic representation of three initial stages of possible emotional reactions to receiving 'bad news' that occur before re-organisation, see Figure 2.2.

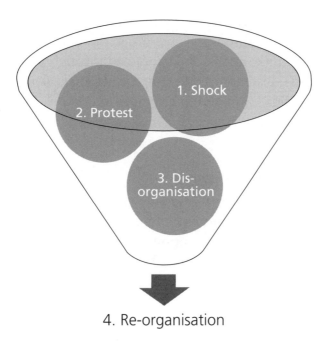

4. Re-organisation

Figure 2.2 A diagrammatic representation of the three initial stages of potential emotional reactions to receiving bad news that occur before re-organisation

It is salient that the information issued is paced in small amounts of clearly stated and uncluttered facts. It is also important not to overload the woman with information in one bite, or confusion and cognitive overloading may occur. Allow time for the woman to go through her 'potential emotional reaction set' before formulating questions she wants to ask during the shock and disbelief stage. It is best not to follow the initial 'bad news' with an information avalanche that is unlikely to be absorbed. Until re-organisation has occurred, stick to the significant points and answer questions that are repeated. Also, reiterate what is necessary as many times as is requested to help facilitate progression to the re-organisation stage.

It is a difficult time for all, professionals included, with those involved requiring to overcome awkwardness that relates to the childbearing woman's grief. In response, accommodate silences and do not feel compelled to fill gaps in the conversation. Show an empathic disposition and encourage the woman to talk when she is ready. Empathy may be expressed through verbal or physical signs. Listen and take a non-judgemental approach. No pressure should be applied in attempts to compel the woman or family to talk. Have respect for individual reactions and coping strategies.

2.2 INITIATING CONVERSATION

It can be really difficult to know where to start. Having the right words is not as important as having a caring presence and being willing to dance attendance upon the bereaved couple. What follows are some ideas that may help the midwife share this journey with the woman and which will optimise time spent together. There is no quick fix to grief and carers cannot fast-track pain. Health and social care professionals need to learn to accept that psychological processes are as they are designed to be. It may be helpful to give the woman a journal in which she can record her thoughts, feelings and memories. This can provide support to the woman as she writes. Also the record can be used to reflect back in years to come on the enduring memory of this grief experience. Some guidelines for a series of conversations follow.

GETTING TO KNOW EACH OTHER

As with all relationships, health and social care professionals need to earn the right for childbearing women to share their grief with them. Building trust is crucial. It may be helpful for them to share a little of themselves with the couple to initiate some connections.

SHARING MEMORIES

It can be helpful to ask the woman to share memories of special things about her pregnancy. These memories could be written in the journal for keepsake. If relevant, ask if the couple would like to peruse photographs that have been taken of their baby and together create meaningful stories to tell. Never force this issue.

As an alternative, the woman can take the photographs in a sealed envelope home with her. Memory jars are another way of creating a meaningful picture of the event and attempting to continue a bond that has been established while the baby was *in utero*.

TELLING THE STORY

Telling the story is a crucial element of support the professional can offer to the woman. It may be the only opportunity she ever has to tell her story to someone who is prepared to listen and fully understands the complexity of her circumstances. The professional can commence the story by asking the woman what life was like before she lost the pregnancy or the baby died. It can be useful to ask her to write or draw her story.

TALKING ABOUT DIFFICULT FEELINGS

Being able to understand that difficult feelings are a normal part of the grieving process can be helpful for the childbearing woman – to know that she is not going mad and that pain, anger, guilt and relief are all acceptable ways to feel when one has lost a baby. This approach can create relief in itself. The carer needs to recognise that the woman will display an array of behavioural changes, with her/his role to provide support absent of judgement. There may be displays of angry behaviour directed at hospital staff. Often this is an outward expression of the woman's inner turmoil. Just expressing understanding that anger is normal is sometimes all that is needed. There are helpful ways to explore difficult feelings. Again, writing in a journal can be cathartic. It may also be helpful to identify what triggers anger and 'pushes buttons'. Sometimes the smaller issues are key and it may be possible to remove them from the environment. Drawing an anger scale may also be useful (see Figure 2.3).

There are many other activities for exploring feelings. For example, visual activities for working with anger and discussing difficult feelings can initiate great conversations.

I feel angry.

Strongly agree	Agree	Neither agree nor disagree	Disagree	Strongly disagree
1	2	3	4	5

Figure 2.3 Anger scale

TALKING ABOUT WHAT HELPS AND DISCUSSING COPING STRATEGIES

Ask the woman what helps her when she feels upset. She may choose to make a list. It may be helpful to listen to music, eat a favourite food, go for a walk and/or look at photographs and mementos. Each person has different coping strategies, and what helps one woman may hinder another. It may also be facilitative to encourage the woman to channel her energies into something positive. For example, exercise releases mood-enhancing hormones.

THINKING ABOUT HOPE FOR THE FUTURE

Women require encouragement to think positively about the future. Regardless of the fact that her baby has died, she can attempt to make the future as she would like it to be. It is important to help her appreciate that she does have some control over her future. The past is behind and out of her control, but she can make her own life choices about the future. It may be helpful for her to write down some of her hopes for a future in a journal. This conversation can be a special time for reflection and can be commemorated by lighting a candle in remembrance of the baby who died. In the future, candles can again be used as reminders, which the family light on special days. A balloon release can also be special. A helium balloon of a significant colour and a written message on paper attached before release can be most therapeutic. Special days, such as anniversaries and imagined birthdays, can be commemorated with such rituals.

BODY LANGUAGE

It is important for maternity care providers to consider their body language when communicating with the woman, her partner and her family. Body language is a form of mental and physical non-verbal communication. It consists of body posture, gestures, facial expressions, and eye movements. Humans send and interpret non-verbal signals almost entirely subconsciously. Human communication consists of 93 per cent body language and paralinguistic cues, with only 7 per cent consisting of actual words (Borg, 2010). Body language provides clues about the attitude and state of mind of the woman. Body language indicates aggression, attentiveness, boredom, relaxed state, pleasure and amusement. This is especially relevant in sensitive situations, such as breaking bad news, since the midwife wants her body language to match what is being communicated verbally. To some extent, what constitutes helpful and unhelpful behaviour is in the eye of the beholder. However, there are certain behaviours that, more often than not, are considered helpful and therefore tend to engender favourable reactions from people. This applies whoever the person is – senior, junior, same-level, clients, patients, friends or relatives. Some examples of helpful body language include (ARC, 2012):

- being open
- being genuine
- making eye contact
- being relaxed and attentive
- smiling where appropriate
- facing the person being addressed.

Unhelpful behaviours are those that hinder the midwife from achieving her/his objectives, or which run the risk of creating a bad impression. What is helpful and unhelpful depends upon circumstances. Nevertheless, there are certain behaviours that tend to engender unfavourable reactions in people the midwife is dealing with. Some examples of unhelpful body language include:

- having a blank expression
- leaning away, arms folded, legs crossed
- using a desk as a barrier
- fidgeting
- hair twirling
- placing hands in front of one's mouth
- talking too loud or too low
- looking bored.

Whilst communicating, it is essential to check for understanding. Clarification may be sought through asking questions. Always respond to questions and consider what follow-up would be appropriate and helpful. This is dependent upon the situation and individual needs of the woman, partner and family. Before closure, the maternity care professional needs to make appropriate contact arrangements and provide details about her/himself, other relevant professionals and potential support persons. Ending the consultation can be difficult. What follows are suggestions about how to close a consultation:

1. Agree further plans.
2. Provide time to gather thoughts.
3. Discuss transport home.
4. Ask if the woman wants a significant person contacted to keep her company.
5. Reinforce contacts.
6. Make some physical contact, e.g. shake hands or touch arm.

2.3 FATHERS AND PERINATAL LOSS

Few would deny that a stillbirth is a traumatic and devastating experience for a family to face. Even though both parents are expected to grieve when such a tragedy occurs, they may in fact grieve differently. It is important that the carers involved recognise that reactions and thinking in relation to events may differ between a couple, with stages of response likely to be out of step with each other. Consequently, it is important to have a discussion

---

Activity 5

Case scenario

You are the professional working on the antenatal ward and have just admitted Fiona, who is a primigravida at 28 week's gestation. Fiona has been transferred into the maternity unit from a rural hospital. From the referral information you are aware that there are concerns about fetal wellbeing and growth. She has been transferred to your unit for more in-depth screening. Fiona is alone and unaccompanied by her partner, and is keen to get in touch with him. She is unaware of the suspected clinical findings. As you conduct a routine cardiotocograph (CTG) trace, Fiona starts to ask questions about her baby and the CTG findings. It is now mid-evening and the doctor is not due to visit until tomorrow.

How will you initially manage this situation?

....
....
....
....
....
....

What ongoing care will you provide for Fiona?

....
....
....
....
....
....

---

with the couple surrounding the issue of each partner allowing the other to grieve in their own individual way. There is no right or wrong approach, but permission to grief in their own manner is a gift that should be granted. Bereavement counsellors often call this difference in timing between mother's and father's 'incongruent grieving'. In addition to dissimilar patterns of progress through the stages of grieving, there is the intensity of the bond between each parent and their infant, which may also differ. For the childbearing woman, bonding is often more instantaneous, evident and passionate right from the start. Her relationship with the future infant more often starts from the time of conception and is forged through meeting her baby's physiological needs whilst inside her and once born. In contrast, due to absence of physical contact with his future child, the father more often forms his attachment through fantasising about their future relationship and what that will entail, e.g. football, fishing trips, graduations etc.

In contemporary society, certain factors may influence a father's attachment to his infant; for example, presence at the birth and viewing the event as a positive experience, or becoming a 'house husband' and fundamentally being the primary care provider to the child. In essence, intensity of bond is influenced by the amount of physical contact, types of experience (positive/negative) and emotional investment in fantasies about future relationships with the unborn child.

What will also affect the way a father grieves is cultural expectations of anticipated behaviour and acceptable responses. In most societies, the man is expected to be the 'strong one' whose main role is to support his grieving partner. That is, the forever practical one who carries out essential tasks. In contrast, the woman is supported to openly express her grief. As a man, he may also believe that open displays of grieving reveal weakness and as such, should be suppressed. In society, the focus tends to place the woman at the centre of attention, with the father sometimes forgotten in the process. It is imperative that staff caring for the couple at this time encourage the father to express his emotions and impress upon him that he is of equal importance in the proceedings. This will involve speaking to both parents directly and asking for separate opinions about how events are to progress. It is important to encourage the childbearing woman to hear and accept her partner's opinions, which may entail both agreement and disagreement with her point of view. Where possible, it is important to accommodate both parents' wishes, either individually or together, and/or encourage the couple to find mutual resolve in the decisions they make. Carers must ensure that the father is not seen as the 'second-class mourner'.

In essence, the father must be afforded his right of passage to grieve. He must not be ignored, neglected or abandoned emotionally. Repression of grief may turn the wheels in motion for a pathological grief process to ensue. Consequences of neglect in expressing grief may result in difficulties with forming attachments to future pregnancies. The father's emotions should not be hidden beneath strata of conscientiousness, responsibility and dependability, otherwise he may erupt with disobliging bursts of negative emotion. Carers, families, friends and work colleagues must encourage both parents to verbalise their thoughts and emotions, with stereotypes and societal templates of male expectations abandoned. Explain to him that he is entitled to his grief and help him find ways to resolve his emotions. One method of encouragement is to ask him to label his underlying emotions and talk about his thoughts. It may be very helpful to provide the father with a booklet to encourage a positive grieving journey.

The Stillbirth and Neonatal Death Society (SANDS) publishes a catalogue of support leaflets with information for mothers, fathers, children, grandparents, family members and friends. These booklets and leaflets are listed below and can be ordered through the online SANDS shop: http://www.uk-sands.org/ Publications/Support-and-information-leaflets.html

LEAFLETS
Mainly for Fathers provides information and support for recently bereaved fathers.
About the Other Children explains how children may perceive the loss of their sibling and provides advice about what others can do to help them cope.
For Family and Friends: How You Can Help explains common reactions of bereaved parents and explains how others may help them cope with their grief.
The Loss of Your Grandchild has been written specifically for grieving grandparents.

Sexual Problems following a Stillbirth acknowledges this sensitive area following the death of a baby.

The Next Pregnancy: Guidance for Parents covers topics such as when to try for a new baby after a previous perinatal loss, being pregnant and how to cope with emotions when the new baby arrives.

BOOKLETS

Saying Goodbye to Your Baby This booklet for parents was first published by SANDS in the 1980s. It has been updated and rewritten, drawing on the experiences and insights of parents who have lost one or more babies. The booklet covers the majority of information that newly bereaved parents may find helpful in the first few days and in the longer term, post-loss. The booklet deals with emotions and practical matters. In addition, family members, friends and health professionals may also find this booklet helpful for gaining understanding of parents' experiences and the issues that may be important for them.

Footprints Is a SANDS national newsletter that is published three times a year and contains a broad range of news and articles about loss, including a section dedicated to personal experiences of bereaved parents and their families.

CONCLUSION

The objective of this chapter is to discuss sensitive and supportive processes involved in delivering bad news to childbearing women, partners and families. Bearing in mind that delivering bereavement care is a holistic process that involves psychological, social, spiritual and physical care, it is important that we not only address psychosocial components, but also describe practical aspects of delivering bereavement care within the maternity unit. One method of doing this is to write down clearly step-by-step information in a protocol that professionals can follow when a perinatal loss occurs. In this way, it can be assured that no essential step in the process is omitted.

Chapter 3 concerns itself with these functional matters through listing relevant activities in protocols and checklists that are to be followed and signed by maternity unit staff when managing an infant loss within a UK maternity unit. Although this workbook is UK-centric, it would be an impossible task to address every society worldwide. Each country has its own unique legal, cultural and social system for managing perinatal death and loss, and it is the business of educators and professionals within each individual society to outline their own duties on how bereavement procedures should be managed.

3

Procedures categorised on a bereavement protocol

Learning objective addressed

On completion of Chapter 3 the reader should be able to:

3. Critically appraise the procedures categorised on a bereavement protocol.

3.1 PROTOCOLS FOR CARING FOR WOMEN WHO HAVE EXPERIENCED LATE FETAL LOSS OR STILLBIRTH

A protocol should tackle seven essential aspects of bereavement care:

1. The care given to parents should be responsive to their individual needs and feelings.
2. Parents require information.
3. Communication with parents should be clear, sensitive and honest.
4. Parents should be treated with respect and dignity.
5. Parental loss should be recognised and acknowledged. Their experience and feelings should be validated.
6. Parents need time to adjust to their loss.
7. All those involved in the care of bereaved parents should have access to support.

Activity 6

Maternity care professionals can address the essential aspects of bereavement care. For example:

- The care given to parents should be responsive to their individual needs and feelings.
- A care plan could be developed that asks specific questions about the couples desires in relation to their management whilst in the maternity unit and post-discharge.

Generate six ideas about ways that midwives can deliver bereavement care in relation to the following principles:

1. Parents require information:

   ....
   ....
   ....

2. Communication with parents should be clear, sensitive and honest:

   ....
   ....
   ....

3. Parents should be treated with respect and dignity:

   ....
   ....
   ....

4. Parents' loss should be recognised and acknowledged. Their experience and feelings should be validated:

   ....
   ....
   ....

5. Parents need time to adjust to their loss:

   ....
   ....
   ....

6. All those involved in the care of bereaved parents should have access to support:

   ....
   ....
   ....

THE AIMS AND OBJECTIVES OF A BEREAVEMENT PROTOCOL

The aims and objectives of a bereavement protocol are as follows:

1. Provide an environment suitable to meet individual needs of the woman and her family following a stillbirth or late fetal loss.
2. Support staff in providing individual family needs.
3. Give essential information to the woman and her family to enable them to make informed choices in relation to subsequent arrangements.
4. Ensure that care provided is evidence-based.
5. Ensure effective prompt communication exists between healthcare professionals and voluntary group members who are providing the bereavement care.

The following are exemplars of protocols designed to guide maternity professionals on management of women who have experienced loss (Tables 3.1–3.11):

> *Notes:*
> - Anticardiolipin/lupus antibodies should not be performed until eight weeks post-pregnancy as doing this earlier can affect the value.
> - Infection screen is not always routinely performed. It is usually only carried out if there is a particular suspicion.
> - Maternal and paternal genetics tests not necessarily routine and only carried out if required. Often done at follow-up after three miscarriages.
> - Blood bottles are not the same in every health board area. Remember to familiarise yourself with local requirements.

CHECKLIST PROCEDURES

It is usual to have a bereavement pack that contains all protocols and checklists to keep maternity professionals on track when caring for a woman/her partner and family who have experienced a late fetal loss or stillbirth.

Activity 7

Maternity care professionals need to address the objectives of a bereavement protocol. Here is an example of a protocol and how directives can be achieved:

- Provide an environment suitable to meet individual needs of the woman and family following a stillbirth or late fetal loss.
- An environment suitable for a grieving couple could consist of a private room with double bed, comfortable chairs, private bathroom, internet access, television, open visiting and privacy from childbearing women who have had successful outcomes and have healthy crying babies.

Now generate four more ideas about ways in which maternity professionals can address the objectives of a bereavement protocol:

1. Support staff in providing individual family needs:

   ....
   ....
   ....

2. Give essential information to the woman and her family to enable them to make informed choices in relation to subsequent arrangements:

   ....
   ....
   ....

3. Ensure that care provided is evidence-based:

   ....
   ....
   ....

4. Ensure effective, prompt communication exists between healthcare professionals and voluntary group members who are providing the bereavement care:

   ....
   ....
   ....

Table 3.1 Protocol of how to manage a woman who has experienced a late fetal loss or stillbirth prior to delivery

1. Medical staff should confirm diagnosis and the woman should be provided with an informed choice about place of delivery. Gestational age may influence the decision about where the woman should deliver.
2. The woman and her family should be welcomed to a family room within the maternity unit by a named midwife ascribed to undertake her care. Members of the appropriate community team should be informed and continuity of care arranged. Time should be provided for questions to be asked and answered.
3. The process of induction should be discussed and a suitable time arranged. This may be immediate or delayed, depending on maternal wellbeing and family wishes.
4. The woman's consultant obstetrician and GP should be informed of her admission to the unit. The antenatal clinic should be notified so that forthcoming scans and appointments can be cancelled.
5. Maternal wellbeing should be assessed, i.e. TPR and BP. Results may influence time of induction.
6. Spiritual guidance should be offered and arranged on request.
7. Following explanation and consent, maternal blood specimens should be collected.
8. Privacy must be afforded at all times.
9. The induction process should commence when appropriate.
10. Care of the woman should continue on an individualised basis and according to her needs. This should include hydration and nutrition.
11. Immediate post delivery care should be discussed with the parents. Decisions require to be made about desire to hold baby, take photographs and post mortem (PM). Discussion should take place with the parents regarding funeral wishes and appropriate forms to be completed:
    - Burial form completed (hospital burial/private burial)
    - Cremation form completed
    If the family opt to have a hospital arranged funeral, the completed forms should be taken to the appropriate office. Parents will be forwarded details of the funeral.
12. When caring for parents following pregnancy loss or death of a baby, the unit checklists should be utilised.

Table 3.2 Protocol of how to manage a woman who has experienced a late fetal loss or stillbirth following delivery

1. Parents should be given time and confidence to see and hold their baby and take photographs if they wish.
2. Photographs should be taken using the unit's digital camera and printed out. If parents do not wish to have copies of the photographs, they should be placed in a sealed envelope and securely stapled to the mother's case notes.
3. A memory box should be offered to the parents. Hand/footprints and a lock of hair are obtained and placed in a memory card. The unit's remembrance book and a church service should be discussed with parents.
4. Parents should be asked if they wish to have their baby bathed and, if appropriate, asked whether they want to be involved. This will depend on the condition of the baby and the extent of maceration. The bathing process should be carried out using cool water.
5. The baby should be examined for abnormalities. If any are identified they should be documented.
6. Appropriate skin, cardiac blood, placental swabs and samples should be collected in accordance with the checklist. In babies of a very young gestational age, it may be difficult to identify sex from genitalia alone. If this is the case, advise parents that further investigations will confirm sex.
7. The baby should be weighed, measured and labelled with two name-bands.
8. The baby should ideally be dressed in personal clothing. Parents may wish to supply this. Where appropriate, parents may wish to dress, or help dress, their baby.
9. Parents should be given the opportunity to have their baby blessed and/or named by a representative of their faith community or the hospital chaplain. Parents can create a personalised funeral for their baby, whatever their beliefs or faith. This may be discussed prior to delivery.
10. The opportunity to have a post mortem (PM) performed should be discussed with the parents. Consent must be obtained.

Table 3.2 continued

11. Once parents are ready, the baby should be transferred to the mortuary with the following forms:

   ■ Confirmation of death
   ■ Removal to mortuary
   ■ Consent to PM (if required).

   Parents should be advised that they can arrange to see their baby again if they wish.

12. If the baby was stillborn (>24 weeks), a stillbirth certificate needs to be completed. This form is taken to the registrar who will record the death. If the baby was born alive, but then died, a neonatal death certificate needs to be completed (regardless of the baby's gestation). Both the birth and death certificates need to be registered.

13. The Confidential Enquiry into Maternal and Child Health (CEMACH) form should be completed and forwarded to the designated co-ordinator.

14. With maternal consent, a teardrop sticker should be applied to the main hospital notes.

15. If the mother is rhesus negative, administration of Anti-D should be arranged if required.

16. Checklists should be completed. If the woman wishes to go home before checklists are completed, omissions need to be communicated to the community team and outstanding tasks documented clearly.

17. The mother should be seen by her own consultant or the on-call consultant for labour ward prior to discharge.

18. It is acceptable for the parents to request to take their baby home for 24 hours after the PM.

19. An appointment should be made with the appropriate office to discuss arrangements and for collection of the necessary documents and certificates.

20. The mother should be allowed home as soon as her medical condition allows.

21. An eight-week follow-up appointment with the named obstetrician and specialist midwife should be made. Test results should be available for discussion on this date.

22. The woman should be given all the necessary contact telephone numbers prior to discharge.

Table 3.2 continued

23. The mother/parents/family should be made aware of counselling services.
24. Staff should be made aware of the employee's counselling service.
25. Explain details of the unit's memorial service for bereaved parents. The chaplainry holds regular memorial services in collaboration with the maternity unit and/or local Stillbirth and Neonatal Death Society (SANDS). These services are tailored to meet the needs of both religious and non-religious bereaved parents.

These guidelines cannot anticipate all possible circumstances and exist only to provide general guidance on clinical management to midwives.

Table 3.3 Checklist 1: Essential communication in bereavement care

Woman informed of death by:

.... Date....................

Partner informed of death by:

.... Date....................

On-call consultant obstetrician informed by:

.... Date....................

Woman's own consultant informed by:

.... Date....................

Team midwife informed by phone:

.... Date....................

GP informed by phone by:

.... Date....................

Health visitors informed by phone by:

.... Date....................

Social worker informed (if applicable) by:

.... Date....................

Antenatal clinic informed by phone by:

.... Date....................

Table 3.4 Checklist 2: maternal investigations

The following specimens should be obtained as soon as possible after fetal demise has been diagnosed and preferably before delivery of the baby:

1. High vaginal swab (prior to delivery if possible)
2. Mid-stream specimen of urine (white-topped bottle)
3. Endocrine screen (grey-topped bottle – 2 mls of blood required)
    ■ HbA1C
    ■ random blood sugar
4. Thyroid function tests (yellow-topped bottle – 3.5 mls of blood required)
    ■ liver function
    ■ bile acids
5. Urea and electrolytes (yellow-topped bottle – 3.5 mls of blood required)
6. Immunological tests (red-topped bottle – 10 mls of blood required)
    ■ anticardiolipin/lupus antibodies (8+ weeks post-loss)
7. Thrombophilia screen (blue-topped bottle – 3.5 mls of blood required)
    ■ lupus, protein S and protein C at six weeks post-natal
8. Haematological tests
    ■ FBC (purple-topped bottle – 3 mls of blood required)
    ■ group & save>
    ■ rhesus antibodies> (pink-topped bottle – 6 mls of blood required)
    ■ kleihauer>
    ■ clotting studies (blue-topped bottle – 3.5 mls).
9. Genetics screen (green-topped bottle)
    ■ Chromosomes
10. Alpha-feto protein (red-topped bottle – 10 mls of blood required)
11. Infection screen (red-topped bottle – 6 mls of blood required)
    ■ TORCH screen
    ■ toxoplasmosis
    ■ rubella
    ■ cytomegalovirus
    ■ herpes simplex
    ■ parvovirus
    ■ listeria
    ■ VDRL

Table 3.5 Checklist 3: fetal investigations

It is important that the following samples are taken from the deceased baby:

1. Baby details:
   - weight
   - length
   - head circumference
   - sex of baby (male/female/uncertain – confirm by PM and/or DNA).

2. In suspected/confirmed cases of fetal abnormality only:
   - skin sample taken at post mortem (full depth 0.5 cm into a dry sterile pot and covered with saline)

3. Cord (2–3 cm taken as near to fetal insertion point as possible (put into a dry sterile pot and cover with saline)

4. Placenta/membrane/cord from as near to insertion point in the placenta as possible (put into a dry sterile pot and cover with saline)

5. Placenta (if consent for PM, placenta is sent with baby in a pot with formalin)

In all cases a small piece of placenta is sent to microbiology in a dry pot. If not for PM, remainder of placenta goes to histopathology in a pot with formalin.

Table 3.6 Checklist 4: post mortem (PM)

Decision to have PM investigation discussed by:	Yes/No
....	
Signature...	Date....................

If baby having PM:

1.	PM leaflet given to parents.	Yes/No
2.	Obtain parents consent on consent form.	Yes/No
3.	Appropriate office informed.	Yes/No
4.	Inform mortuary of date and time of arrival.	Yes/No
5.	Inform parents that results will be issued in approximately eight weeks.	Yes/No
6.	Baby is sent to mortuary accompanied by:	
	■ consent to PM form	Yes/No
	■ photocopy of case notes	Yes/No
7.	Doctor decides if additional tests are required, e.g. genetic screening.	Yes/No

Table 3.7 Checklist 5: provision of emotional and spiritual support

Emotional support provided by:.................................... Yes/No

Signed .... Date...................

1.	Parents held baby	Yes/No
2.	Photographs taken with polaroid camera	Yes/No
3.	Photographs given to parents/stored in notes	Yes/No
4.	Photographs taken with digital camera	Yes/No
5.	Parents taken photographs with own camera	Yes/No
6.	Mementos given	Yes/No
7.	Memory box given	Yes/No
8.	Memory card given	Yes/No
9.	Hand and footprints taken	Yes/No
10.	Lock of hair taken	Yes/No
11.	Name band given	Yes/No
12.	Spiritual support	Yes/No
13.	Baby named/blessed/baptised	Yes/No
14.	Naming/blessing/baptism certificate given	Yes/No
15.	Seen by chaplain	Yes/No
16.	SANDS information leaflets provided	Yes/No

Table 3.8 Checklist 6: parents request to take the baby home

Discuss parents' requests to take baby home with consultant obstetrician.

Parents can take the baby home if there is no PM being undertaken or after PM has been carried out (not *before* PM).

A stillbirth certificate must be completed prior to taking the baby home.

Parents should be advised:
- that in the event of a PM there may be leakage from the restoration suturing site
- to keep their baby in a cool room
- to exclude pets from the room.

The baby should be transported home in a crib.

A letter explaining the situation should be handed to the parents in case of police interest.

Baby should be returned to the hospital mortuary within 24 hours of departure.

Table 3.9 Checklist 7: funeral arrangements

Funeral arrangements discussed by:	Yes/No
Signed	Date....................

Do family wish to have:
- a burial?   Yes/No
- a cremation?   Yes/No

Do family wish to have:
- a hospital burial?   Yes/No
- a private cremation?   Yes/No

Parents informed they can choose to attend/not attend hospital burial.	Yes/No
If family decide to attend hospital funeral, inform general office.	Yes/No
If specimens are to be returned to the baby, funeral may be delayed.	Yes/No
Parents offered contact details of hospital chaplain for further information about what cremation/funeral involves and experiences of other bereaved parents.	Yes/No

Parents should be encouraged to take their time before making decisions about funeral arrangements. Choices should be outlined orally before discharge and also given on paper. Ask parents to make contact with the maternity unit when finalised. Provide contact numbers and addresses.

Telephone number...	Yes/No
Email address...	Yes/No

Comments...
....
....
....
....

Table 3.10 Checklist 8: Forms to be completed

Forms completed by: .... Yes/No

Signed .... Date ....

The following forms may need to be completed:

Confirmation of death form completed	Yes/No
If for PM, consent to PM form completed	Yes/No
Consent for removal of tissue samples (on the PM Form)	Yes/No
Removal to mortuary form completed	Yes/No
If born alive, then died, neonatal death certificate	Yes/No
Burial form completed:	
■ hospital burial	Yes/No
■ private burial	Yes/No
Cremation form completed (if applicable)	Yes/No
Antenatal clinic notification form completed	Yes/No
Delivery details entered on computer	Yes/No
Clinical incident form completed	Yes/No
Suspected congenital anomaly form	Yes/No
Stillbirth certificate completed	Yes/No
Neonatal death certificate completed (if applicable)	Yes/No
Parents informed of registration procedure	Yes/No

Table 3.11 Checklist 9: discharge procedures

Discharge procedures carried out by: ....

Signed .... Date...................

Baby

Ensure two name-bands fastened to baby prior to mortuary transfer	Yes/No
If parents did not want to see their baby, offer the opportunity again before discharge	Yes/No
Shroud/sheet ticket completed and secured to baby	Yes/No
Wrap baby appropriately before transfer to mortuary	Yes/No
Copied forms completed and sent to mortuary with baby	Yes/No
Removal to mortuary form signed by transferring porter	Yes/No

Mother

Mother's notes completed	Yes/No
Teardrop sticker applied to notes	Yes/No
Follow-up appointment discussed	Yes/No
Drugs discussed, prescribed and discharge pack given	Yes/No
Seen by on-call consultant before discharge	Yes/No
Remembrance book discussed with parents	Yes/No
Inform GP by phone of mother's discharge	Yes/No
Inform community midwife by phone of mother's discharge	Yes/No
Discuss physical care/emotional reactions	Yes/No
Give parents appropriate office contact number	Yes/No
Ensure parents have community midwife's name and number	Yes/No
Arrange postnatal appointment for twelve weeks post delivery	Yes/No

3.2 MANAGING MATERNAL DEATH

When a maternal death occurs, it is a far-reaching and tragic event that resonates throughout the entire maternity unit. It is one of the most challenging and upsetting events that midwives and allied healthcare professionals encounter in their daily work. Consequently, it is salient that staff prepare themselves for experiencing such an event and learn to provide appropriate guidance, advice and support to the deceased woman's partner, family and friends. It is also important that they learn to care for themselves and colleagues who become involved in the incident. In addition to the emotional and social implications of such an event, it is important to outline the practical and essential activities that require to be fulfilled when a maternal death occurs. To provide clarity of understanding, the first task when addressing this sensitive topic is to define precisely categories of the term 'maternal death'.

WHAT IS A MATERNAL DEATH?

Maternal death refers to the death of a woman while pregnant or within 42 days of termination of pregnancy, irrespective of the duration and site of the pregnancy from any cause related to or aggravated by the pregnancy or its management, but not from accidental or incidental causes (WHO, 2010). Classifications of maternal death include:

Direct maternal death
Maternal death resulting from an obstetric complication of pregnancy, labour or the puerperium from interventions, omissions, incorrect treatment, or from a chain of events resulting from any of the above.

Indirect maternal death
Maternal death that results from previous existing disease or disease that developed during pregnancy and which was not due to direct obstetric causes, but which was aggravated by the physiological effects of pregnancy.

Coincidental death
Maternal death that occurs from unrelated causes that occur in
the pregnancy or puerperium, such as an accident.

Late death
Maternal death that occurs between 42 days and one year after
abortion, miscarriage or delivery that is due to direct or indirect
maternal causes.

The key indicator for gauging progress towards achieving a
reduction in the maternal mortality rate is the number of maternal
deaths that occur during a given time period per 100,000 live
births. Many countries monitor the numbers of maternal deaths
with accurate measurements not available in 115 countries due to
inadequate civil registration systems (WHO, 2012).

The Confidential Enquiries into Maternal Deaths (CEMD),
which began in 1957, has been the longest-running clinical audit
in the world (Ngan Kee, 2005). In 2003, CEMD joined with
CESDI (stillbirths and deaths in infancy) and became CEMACH
(Confidential Enquiry into Maternal and Child Health) and was
part of the Royal College of Obstetricians and Gynaecologists
(RCOG). In 2009 it became an independent body known as
CMACE (Centre for Maternal and Child Enquiries). This
triennial report has always maintained the focus of monitoring
and reducing maternal deaths and improving the safety of
childbirth by providing an overview of the numbers and causes of
maternal deaths in the UK. These enquiries, and similar audits in
other countries are used to guide improvements in clinical practice
that can work towards preventing comparable future deaths
(Yentis, 2011). Indeed, since 2003, the CEMACH and CMACE
reports have focused upon saving mothers' lives, which is
reflected in a proactive approach to preventing maternal deaths.
The CEMACH's *Why Mother's Die*, Sixth Report (2004) alerted
health professionals to the fact that the largest cause of indirect
deaths and, indeed, the largest cause of all maternal deaths was
due to psychiatric illness in the period 2000–2002. This shocking
statistic highlighted the impact of maternal death on children and

families and the need for changes in service delivery, especially to more vulnerable women. During that period (2000–2002), 543 children lost their mother due to maternal death, mainly due to suicide (Lewis, 2004), which has huge implications for bereavement care requirements for the remaining family members.

During the period 2006–2008 there were 261 maternal deaths reported in the UK, with 107 categorised as direct and 154 as indirect. The direct death rate decreased from 6.24 per 100,000 maternities in 2003–2005 to 4.6 per 100,000 maternities in 2006–2008.

It is essential that professionals working with childbearing women can effectively manage bereavement events when the periodic maternal death occurs. In general, five direct complications account for more than 70 per cent of maternal deaths worldwide. These include the following approximations of cause:

- haemorrhage (25%)
- infection (15%)
- unsafe abortion (13%)
- eclampsia (9%)
- obstructed labour (8%).

The remaining losses are caused by or associated with diseases such as malaria and AIDS during pregnancy. Whilst these are the central causes of maternal death around the world, the main predisposing factors are mismanagement of events due to unavailable, inaccessible, unaffordable, or poor-quality care and lack of equipment. Maternal death outcome is also detrimental to the social development and wellbeing of around one million children left motherless each year. Consequently, it is the role of maternity and paediatric professionals to help prevent maternal death through providing the information and support that is required to optimise reproductive health, guide childbearing women safely through pregnancy, and care for both her and the newborn infant well into childhood. Throughout the world the vast majority of maternal deaths could be prevented if women had access to:

- quality family planning services
- skilled care during pregnancy, childbirth and the first month post-delivery
- safe abortion services
- effective emergency obstetric services.

Maternal mortality is one of the health indicators that reflect the greatest disparity between people who are rich and poor. The fact that more than 90 per cent of maternal deaths and morbidities occur in developing countries indicates that these supply-constrained settings lack adequate and available resources and health service facilities. The maternal mortality ratio in developing countries is 240 per 100,000 births versus 16 per 100,000 in developed countries, with the World Health Organisation committed to achieving a reduction in present levels of maternal death by three-quarters.

Professionals involved in providing maternity care play a key role in the ongoing CEMD by first recognising that a maternal death has occurred and secondly by ensuring that the appropriate people have been notified. Maternal death may occur in a number of clinical and non-clinical settings and may result from a complication of miscarriage, termination of pregnancy, ectopic pregnancy, cardiac disease, medical disorder, surgical procedure or suicide or an accident. In addition to the vast input of psychosocial management that is involved, what follows is an exemplar of a protocol designed to guide maternity care staff through the myriad of paperwork procedures involved when a maternal death occurs in the UK.

3.3 PROTOCOL DISCUSSION

It is psychologically traumatic to give birth to a stillborn child. The emotional changes experienced by parents are enormous. Several decades ago, stillbirth was normally regarded as a

Table 3.12 Protocol of how to manage a maternal death

1. A maternal death may occur in the community or in a maternity unit or hospital. The responsibility for notifying the *Regional Coordinator* that a maternal death has occurred rests with the consultant, midwife or general practitioner (GP) who has had overall responsibility for the deceased childbearing woman's pregnancy. When the death occurs within one year following the end of a pregnancy, death is notified by the consultant or GP who treated the woman during her final illness. This responsibility may be delegated to the nominated *Maternal Death Co-ordinator*. Information required to be given includes the:

    ■ deceased's name, address, date of birth and date of death
    ■ considered cause of death
    ■ place of death

    (a) When the maternal death occurs within the maternity unit, a *Senior Midwife* or *Supervisor of Midwives* (SoM) is nominated to undertake the role of co-ordinator for the maternal death. If an SoM has not been nominated to act as co-ordinator in accordance with the Midwives' Rules and Code of Practice (NMC, 1998) Code 39, the on-call supervisor must be notified that the maternal death has occurred.
    (b) When the maternal death occurs outside the maternity unit, the person in charge of the hospital department must notify the senior midwife or SoM who is responsible for co-ordinating maternal deaths at the local maternity unit.
    (c) The co-ordinator must ensure that a record of each part of the procedure is maintained. There should be a pack of appropriate forms pre-prepared for such events.

2. A suitable full-time named member of staff should be nominated to support the woman's family and act as its entrusted delegate. This person must ensure that conflicting information is not given by the many people who may become involved.
3. The *consultant* or *consultant on call* must meet as soon as possible with the deceased woman's relatives. The named consultant should speak with the family as soon as is timely possible.

Table 3.12 continued

---

4. The mortuary department attendant is informed of the maternal death and when to expect the deceased woman's arrival.
   (a) The pathologist is organised to undertake a post mortem to confirm cause of death.
   (b) Permission for the post mortem to be conducted is sought from the deceased woman's next of kin. If the cause of death is unknown, the coroner is informed and will order a mandatory post mortem.

6. The case notes and appropriate documentation should be completed, photocopied and secured at the first opportunity. If the coroner decides to hold a hearing about the case, the case notes and documentation must be sent to the coroner's office for appraisal.

7. Risk management processes should be activated and an internal investigation initiated.

8. Staff involved in the case should be offered professional and personal support. This may be provided by the SoM, Hospital Chaplain or a trained person from Human Resources. Services of a trained counsellor must be made available to staff involved for an indefinite period of time post-event.

9. (a) In the event that the fetus has died before its mother, local stillbirth/neonatal death procedures must be followed.
   (b) Removal of the deceased baby from its deceased mother is not a requirement.

10. Relatives should be offered a visit from the hospital chaplain and/or a priest, vicar, rabbi or preacher applicable to their own religious affiliation.

11. The following persons should be notified of the maternal and/or fetal death:
    - Trust Chief Executive Officer
    - Directorate Clinical Director
    - Risk Manager
    - Community Midwife
    - Clinical Managers
    - Government Regional Co-ordinator for maternal deaths
    - General Practitioner
    - Health Visitor
    - Local Supervising Authority (LSA) Officer for Midwifery Supervision.

Table 3.12 continued

12. Arrangements should be made for the woman's family to meet with the consultant for a minimum of one further meeting.
13. The consultant must complete the death certificate. Relatives are asked to deliver this certificate to the *Registrar of Births and Deaths*.
14. In situations where the cause of the maternal death is unknown, the Coroner's Officer (more often a policeman) may insist on accompanying relatives on visits to view the body (bodies) of their deceased loved ones in the mortuary. Sensitive handling and co-ordination will be required in such events.
15. A social worker should be asked to visit if the family's social circumstances are applicable or if a live baby requires care and family support.

non-event (Bourne, 1968). Nowadays, the approach is the reverse. The contemporary view endorses that parents should be confronted with the reality, as this facilitates healthy mourning. This involves the midwife practising the routines outlined in the protocols. Such schedules have limitations, in that staff may inflexibly apply the prescribed steps, stipulating, for example, that all women should hold their stillborn child (Kennel and Traause, 1978). The risk is that checklists and behavioural protocols can produce chronic institutionalisation of bereavement (Leon, 1992).

With reference to parental decision-making following an *in utero* death, Hughes *et al.* (2002) assert that mothers have no clear plan of how to manage their situation, quite simply because they are in shock. Therefore, they usually go along with what they perceive is expected of them, rather than actively making choices that meet their own particular needs. Parents should be given information that will aid their decision-making in both oral and written form. After a period of time has been given to peruse, consider and reflect, they should then be provided with ample opportunity to ask questions and clarify issues (Brown, 1993).

Radestad *et al.* (1996) in a nationwide Swedish population-based epidemiological study concluded that it is advisable to induce delivery as soon as possible post diagnosis of death *in utero*. A calm environment for the woman to spend as much time as she wants with her stillborn infant is beneficial and tokens of remembrance should be collected. The results of the study contradicts the high figures for psychological morbidity previously reported (LaRoche *et al.*, 1984; Nicol *et al.*, 1986; Rowe *et al.*, 1978; Toedter *et al.*, 1988). Zeanah (1989) and Kirkley-Best and Kellner (1982) criticise these studies for their lack of standardised ways of measuring outcome, the lack of a control group and the low precision due to small numbers. Radestad *et al.* (1996) also noted a strong association between waiting more than 24 hours before commencing delivery after the diagnosis of death *in utero* and related anxiety symptoms. Thus, postponing delivery for a length of time can induce unnecessary negative psychological experiences that are difficult to cope with. The optimal interval from diagnosis *in utero* to induction of delivery remains uncertain, but more than 24 hours is too long. Radestad *et al.* (1996) also found that not offering the woman the opportunity to see the infant for as long as she wants, and a lack of tangible tokens of remembrance increase the risks of anxiety and depression.

Minimising such incidents requires skill on the part of the maternity care providers. The woman's expressions of grief and shock may also be accompanied by feelings of pride in her child; therefore the care offered should embrace a meeting and a parting of the infant simultaneously. Confronting mothers of stillborn babies with the reality of the death has been thought to facilitate healthy mourning (Radestad *et al.*, 1996). Rather than enforcing mourning rituals, flexibility should be shown towards the mother's own needs. The notion that, while creating a tranquil atmosphere around the newborn baby post-delivery, maternity care providers should not force the mother to hold, caress or kiss the deceased child. Mothers wishing to engage in activities should be supported, whilst those who wish to abstain should be allowed to do so.

It is psychologically traumatic to give birth to a stillborn child. A stillbirth is often unexpected and happens quickly, and the emotional changes experienced by the parents are enormous. Investigations have reported that 20–30 per cent of women with perinatal loss of a child have appreciable psychiatric long-term morbidity (Barr and Cacciatore, 2008; Kennel and Klaus, 1970; Kroth *et al.*, 2004; Lasker and Toedter, 1991, 2000). Consequently, it is salient for the carers to understand processes of bereavement that enhance positive outcomes and diminish those that are negative.

Many parents will not know what a cremation or funeral involves. Consequently, they will require time to consider potential decisions after being given knowledge from which to make informed choices. For example, burial means that parents have a special place to visit and remember their baby. A hospital burial usually involves the deceased being laid to rest in an area of a cemetery exclusively for babies. Cremation of the baby may involve no ashes to disperse afterwards, unlike what happens with a deceased adult. This situation is dependent upon the type of cremator used and the question needs to be asked in advance of making the decision. It may be important for some parents to visit their intended crematorium or cemetery in advance of their decision. Often graves are elaborately marked, dependent upon local regulations, with parents having to consider what they would want for themselves before deciding to have their baby laid to rest there.

It is a good idea for the maternity unit to keep a folder with pictures of the local baby cemetery and graves held within. Parents may find this helpful whilst deciding. Such viewing may also lessen fear of the unknown for parents on the day of the funeral or cremation. Significant numbers of parents change their mind about attending or not attending the funeral of their baby. As such, they require as much information as possible prior to making an informed choice about funeral arrangements (Kelly, 2007). Attendance or non-attendance at the funeral is an area of personal preference, and parents should never be made to feel obliged to be present. However, once their baby has been buried or cremated, the style in which the ceremony was conducted cannot be reversed. Decisions made have the potential to influence the parents' subsequent grief process. Hence, stressing the importance of giving parents time to think through their decisions about laying their baby to rest, the rituals that take place and marking of the grave are important.

Formal ritual marking, such as blessing, naming and having a funeral for the baby, may empower bereaved parents to feel they have parented their baby in some constructive way in the given set of circumstances (Kelly, 2007). If parents choose to be actively involved in co-creating or personalising rituals, it can work towards them feeling that they are retaining some control. Through choice provision, the parents are afforded a place to be creative in a situation that otherwise they may feel they have failed to create. Such involvement can enhance parental self-worth (ibid.). Rituals can enable parents to act out their relationship with their baby with some dignity and pride (McHaffie, 2001). Examples of rituals may include carrying the coffin into the crematorium or lowering the coffin into the ground. Doing so can create special memories and an association with their baby (Kelly, 2007), which may deepen 'continuing bonds'. (Klass *et al.*,1996). Of course, such actions may not be the choice of all parents. It is important not to make parents feel that they should ritualise the reality of their baby's death in this particular way. Nevertheless, active involvement in informed decision-making regarding the place and type of funeral and the form and content of ritual marking of their baby's short life and death can enable parents to create some meaning and purpose at this time of loss. Being involved in rituals can create constructive memories and give parents something to hold on to and reflect upon for the rest of their lives (Kelly, 2007).

CONCLUSION

The objective of this chapter is to discuss procedures categorised in a bereavement protocol; the purpose of which is to facilitate

Activity 8

A Stillbirth and Neonatal Death Society (SANDS) teardrop sticker may be used to distinguish the notes of a woman whose baby has died both in the time following the death and during subsequent pregnancies. This sticker alerts staff to a previous bereavement and ensures that everyone involved in the care of the woman, partner and family are aware of the loss and do not inadvertently say anything that could augment distress. Teardrop stickers can be used on the GP notes for the mother, the father, siblings and grandparents. Individuals must provide consent before their notes are marked with a teardrop sticker. The label should be placed in a prominent position on the outside cover.

Task
Be creative and design your own teardrop sticker in the space below:

Activity 9

Self-assessment test

1. Classify ten areas of maternity practice that may incur bereavement:

....

....

....

....

2. Differentiate between the meaning of the terms 'loss', 'grief' and 'bereavement':

....

....

....

....

3. Discuss the four dimensions of a childbearing woman's response to a significant loss:

....

....

....

....

4. What are the six essential aspects of bereavement care that a protocol should tackle?

....

....

....

....

5. What are the aims and objectives of a bereavement protocol?

....

....

....

6. Critically discuss the role of checklists within bereavement care:

....

....

....

....

....

....

....

....

....

....

....

....

....

....

professionals with completing their legal and functional requirements. Returning from the practical to the psychological processes surrounding perinatal bereavement, Chapter 4 attempts to provide explanations of ways of understanding how individuals who encounter perinatal loss experience the event psychologically. Many philosophers and psychologists have studied the processes involved and have attempted to capture what is experienced in a formulaic way. Although these occurrences can never be precise, with each individual experience unique, they are an attempt at helping the inexperienced gain experience without having actually taking the voyage themselves. In addition, these models are useful for helping the individual who is experiencing loss to understand their own internal mechanisms of coping with their grief.

4

Models of grieving

Learning objective addressed

On completion of Chapter 4 the reader should be able to:

4. Critically appraise the models of grieving.

In Chapter 1, some aspects of grieving in relation to maternity care provision were considered. In contrast, this chapter looks more closely at the stages of grieving and will provide you with more in-depth perspectives on grief.

4.1 MODELS OF GRIEVING

Grief and grieving theory have tenuous roots in Freud's psychoanalytical theory, but Lindemann (1944) is credited with the first attempt to explain the grieving process. The most well-known work is the classic stages of the grieving process as defined by Kubler-Ross (1969). Kubler-Ross originally applied these stages to people facing death, but later recognised that these could pertain to any form of catastrophic personal loss (e.g. loss of job, income or freedom). Kubler-Ross suggested that the identified stages of grieving could be recognised in many significant life events, such as death of a loved one, divorce, drug addiction, the onset of a disease or chronic illness, an infertility diagnosis, as well as many tragedies and disasters.

Activity 10

Reflect on an episode in your life that has resulted in a sense of loss. This may be due to the loss of a job, being jilted by a boyfriend or the loss of a grandparent.

Write down words that describe your feelings immediately and over time:

....

....

....

Discuss these feelings with reference to the description of the grieving process that follows:

....

....

....

The grieving process, as described by Kubler-Ross, moves through the following five stages:

Denial – Initially the person expresses disbelief that death has occurred. They may feel that the world is a meaningless place and be overwhelmed by events. They are likely to present in a state of shock, but as they begin to accept what has occurred enter the next stage.

Anger – They may feel confused and begin to find blame in everyone around. They may be angry with the midwives and obstetricians who let this happen, with partner and friends, with self and maybe also with God.

Bargaining – They may bargain with self and others and hope that by fulfilling their side of the bargain they will wake up from this nightmare to find it was all a dream. They enter the stage of 'if only' or 'what if' and want to turn back the clock to do things differently in hope of a better outcome.

Depression – They may enter a period of time where they recognise how empty their lives are without the individual who has died. They may feel deeply depressed as they try to come to terms with life without that person.

Acceptance – Eventually the pain of their loss should diminish as they recognise that life must continue. A new pattern of normal life emerges. The person is never forgotten. Memories remain, but these become an accepted part of the new reality.

Although Kubler-Ross (1969) clearly defined these stages, it is essential to recognise that grieving is a very dynamic process that individuals experience to a greater or lesser degree. Not every individual experiences every stage. Reactions to illness, death and loss are as unique as the person experiencing them. Those caring for the bereaved woman must also recognise that individuals may go through the process at different paces and in a different order and may regress to an earlier stage before moving on. Evidence now points towards a more general pattern that fits most of the theories written about the process of grieving. What is important is that carers recognise that the process may manifest differently between individuals.

The immediate reaction to the unfolding event is a temporary defensive mechanism of delaying tactics that aid denial and, inevitability, of the death (Engel, 1961). This enables the individual to prepare emotionally for the reality of loss. Kubler-Ross (1969) identifies this phase as one of *denial*. This reaction has been explained by Jones (1989) in terms of shock, both physiologically and/or psychologically. In the event that denial becomes extreme, it may be classified as a pathological reaction to loss and should be managed appropriately.

After a variable length of time, the individual enters a period of developing awareness of the inevitability of loss or death. During this phase, powerful emotions may be displayed, such as *anger* and expressions of guilt. Wrath may manifest towards any number of individuals who may or may not have been involved in the loss event. Feelings of guilt may relate to unfinished business, to activities carried out during pregnancy or to lack of input into care. Some people find that they are unable to let go of the lost individual, feeling his/her presence nearby, or experience hallucinations such as hearing the baby cry (Mander, 2006). As this phase progresses, the individual may make silent *bargains* to a higher being, such as God, in an attempt to delay or even prevent the imminent loss. However, once it is clear that these tactics are going to be unsuccessful, the grieving individual may enter a period of apathy and despondency, which Bowlby (1961) terms disorganisation.

The next phase is one of full realisation of the loss. Many theorists identify this as a period of profound *depression* (Jones, 1989; Kubler-Ross, 1969). Depression brings with it very real symptoms of psychological distress, which may include sleeplessness, loss of appetite and the inability to concentrate on tasks for a given period of time. This phase can become very protracted.

The final phase is one of resolution. Kubler-Ross (1969) calls this *acceptance* that life must go on. The lost individual becomes a valued, accepted and realistic part of future memories. There is an ongoing debate about whether this includes the severance of emotional bonds (Walter, 1999).

Whilst there are obvious differences between the ways women manifest their grief, in generic terms the underlying processes are the same between the sexes. During the avenue of recovery, it is vitally important that the experiencer establishes a support network and shares events with others who are also deeply affected. During this time, shared activities can help strengthen bonds between family members and friends, and work towards creating constructive memories.

ADDITIONAL MODELS OR THEORIES OF BEREAVEMENT

In addition, researchers have developed several new models or theories to help professionals understand the processes of bereavement. These models serve to facilitate professionals who are involved in supporting the bereaved, by providing a knowledge base from which to practise. With this in mind, a further five bereavement models/theories have been selected to enhance sensitivity of professionals who work with the bereaved.

1. Bowlby's (1961, 1981) theory of attachment

Bowlby (1961, 1981) provides an explanation for the common human tendency to develop strong affectionate bonds to the deceased individual. He views attachment as a reciprocal relationship that results from long-term interactions between an infant and his or her parents. Bowlby proposes that grief is an inherent response to separation and that the grieving process follows a predictable orderly pattern of response to the loss. The initial shock that results in numbness can last for days, especially when a death is sudden. This initial reaction normally proceeds to intense grief, which may be accompanied by physical symptoms, such as chest tightness, shortness of breath, loss of appetite and/or insomnia. Lack of concentration, restlessness, feelings of isolation, loneliness, anger, guilt and fear may also be in accompaniment. Anger expressed depends on the individual's circumstances, with guilt often associated with self-recrimination for things done or not done. When these feelings are suppressed, the bereaved woman may exhibit irritation. Fear may manifest as insecurity, a desire to escape from reality, or as anxiety. These responses become irregular when they induce panic attacks and/or normal living is disrupted.

2. Worden's (1983, 1991) tasks for the bereaved

Worden (1983, 1991) described grief as a process and not a state, with people requiring to work through their reactions in order to make a complete adjustment to their loss. Bereavement is considered to consist of four overlapping tasks that the bereaved person requires to work through whilst adjusting to changes in circumstances, roles, status and social identity. These tasks are completed when the bereaved person has integrated the loss into their life and let go of their emotional attachment to the deceased individual. Once the bereaved person has completed their tasks of mourning, they are free to invest in the present and the future.

3. Stroebe and Schut's (1999) dual process model

Stroebe and Schut (1999) suggest that avoiding grief may be both helpful and detrimental, depending upon circumstances. Whilst prior models centred on loss, the dual process model acknowledges that expressing and controlling feelings are important. The dual process model introduces the idea that the bereaved individual oscillates between focusing on the loss of the pregnancy and baby (loss orientation) and avoiding that focus (restoration orientation). *Loss orientation* encompasses grief work, whilst *restoration orientation* involves dealing with secondary losses that result from the death. For example, an older widow may have to deal with finances and house maintenance that her deceased husband previously dealt with. Both *loss orientation* and the *restoration orientation* are necessary for future adjustments to be made.

4. Klass et al.'s (1996) continuing bonds theory

Klass *et al.* (1996) challenged conventional thinking that the purpose of grieving was the reconstitution of an autonomous individual who could leave the deceased behind and form future attachments. This requires bonds to be broken with the deceased infant. Instead, Klass *et al.* propose that the purpose of grieving is to maintain a bond with the deceased individual, which is compatible with other, new and continuing relationships.

5. Families making sense of death theory

Most models of grief deal with individuals who have experienced loss. However, more often, death affects the family as a whole, with the loss holding different meaning for each member. Families in which there are fragile relationships, secrets and members who hold differing belief systems may have greater difficulty adjusting to the loss, in contrast to those who have frequent contact, rituals and willingness for each member to share their feelings.

In summary, most models of grief suggest that the bereaved person requires to engage and work through their loss in order for life to be reordered and regain meaning. Most health and social care professionals are familiar with the stage theories that identify cognitive, social and emotional factors (e.g. Kubler-Ross). In addition, Worden's (1983) tasks of bereavement provide a framework to guide grief work, while the dual-process model demonstrates the need to deal with both the primary loss and secondary stressors (Stroebe and Schut, 1999). It is important to acknowledge that the bereaved childbearing woman and family do not need to forget and leave their deceased baby behind. Instead, they can integrate them into their future lives through continuing to bond with them through memories. It is also important to identify tensions between family members and assess how each person is influencing one another's adaptation process and what the loss means to each of them. It is also important to acknowledge that there are no rights or wrongs in relation to how to grieve. No model of grieving is recommended above another, as all have mechanisms that may be helpful towards aiding understanding of the bereavement process and the processes involved in adaptation to loss.

4.2 CULTURAL DIVERSITY AND THE ROLE OF RITUAL IN RELATION TO LOSS

Rituals afford worth and systems to grieving. Instigating discussions about rituals and their timing are important elements for the carer of a bereaved family. Throughout history, civilisations have used rituals to signpost critical life events at both a social and personal level. Marriage ceremonies and birthday celebrations are examples of rituals that are conducted across the majority of cultures. Although rituals vary between race, religions and cultures, they offer organisation and assist articulation of emotions for individuals who are grieving. That is, they systematise a structured way to bid farewell to a treasured being and begin the healing journey. Rituals acknowledge the reality of death, provide social support, encourage expression of emotions, and help with converting the relationship between the childbearing woman and her deceased from future to past. Each perinatal death marks the commencement of grief work for families and creates opportunities for use of ceremonies. Whether rituals of transition are sacred or secular, they convey significance that expands beyond the event itself. Anthropologists study these symbolic rites of passage, which consist of events that are repeated over and over again to emotionally manage specified situations. Organisation and empathetic cues organise behaviours associated with such specific events. Out of repeated behaviours rituals become established, and from these, ways of life develop.

Ordinarily, death marks the final transition from life on this earth. In contrast, a perinatal death encompasses a life that has never really commenced. Within the maternity unit this makes it a unique event.

Lack of recognition by the external world experienced by some women after a perinatal death can predispose them to delayed or extended bereavement (Kavanaugh *et al.*, 2004). Parents mourn for their loss, but also for the demise of an anticipated future. Failure of others to acknowledge the magnitude of grief and provide lack of support can direct a complicated grief process. Ritual can deliberate and focus action designed to declare a pregnancy loss or stillbirth. Whatever ritual is undertaken, it must be meaningful to the childbearing woman, with the use of symbols, words or concrete items creating meaning. These Items are precious reminders of the ritual of goodbye. Rituals offer a means of recognising the extent of loss and provide opportunity to articulate emotions. It is important to acknowledge that not all women will want the rituals that are offered, and it is imperative not to criticise those who reject such suggestions.

It is the caregiver's responsibility to act as a guide and provide empathetic support to the grieving woman and her family. Within this role, activating rituals is key. Individualising care involves unearthing the childbearing woman's perceived values and needs in relation to how events surrounding the death of her baby are managed. In other words, personalise meaning-making within the family's cultural context. For example, in Mexico it is custom for the family to remain close to their deceased loved one's body and

CASE STUDY

The maternity care providers role in participation in the ritual of baptism.

You are a midwife in the delivery suite of a maternity unit. The admissions midwife calls to inform you that a childbearing woman at 23 gestational weeks is in the second stage of labour. Willow and her partner Arnold arrive and within five minutes she delivers a baby girl called Melody who is allocated an APGAR score of 1 and resuscitation is attempted. In full awareness that death is imminent you baptise the baby in keeping with how you were taught in college.

Discussion
This case study exemplifies the crucial role of ritual. However, there are a few issues that must be discussed. Were the midwife to be asked about intention for undertaking the christening, it would probably be that she was thinking about the parents' needs. But the intention omitted to identify what the parents in fact needed. That is, the parents' wishes for their baby in this particular situation. It is possible that they are non-Christian and have no requirement for the action you took.

■ What aspects of parental need did the midwife ignore?

....
....
....
....
....

■ List questions you would ask to open conversations with Willow and Arnold to explore their belief systems surrounding baptism.

....
....
....
....
....
....
....

not leave it for some time after death. This involves the couple staying with their infant's body until it is released for post mortem and forwarded to the funeral director. A plan of action to best honour the woman's beliefs requires to be formulated.

QUESTIONS FOR THE CARER AND THE WOMAN

- Help me understand what we can do to help you and your family cope with your baby's death.
- Are there any family customs you would like us to enact?
- How would you like events to unfold?
- What is important for you to remember?
- What traditions would you and your family like accommodated?

In a case akin to the aforementioned, it is important to explain that the baby's body can remain with the couple until a funeral director has been selected, but beforehand, at some point, it will be required to go to the morgue. They could be offered the opportunity to accompany their baby on its journey to the morgue to formulate a picture in their head of where it will be until a funeral director has been selected. Also, they should be welcome to revisit as often as they feel they require. Staff empathy could be expressed through sending cards, attending the funeral and, post-discharge, through telephone calls. Co-creation of rituals may involve transforming a routine procedure, such as discharge, into an explicit ritual; for example, asking the couple if they would like you to play a specific piece of music as they exit the maternity unit.

TAKING THE BABY HOME

Some parents may decide that they want to take their deceased baby home or to a place of special meaning for a short while. There is legally no challenge to this undertaking unless a post mortem has been ordered immediately by the coroner. It is a good idea to give the parents a form that states that they have been authorised by the hospital to undertake this activity, just in case they are stopped by authority and questioned. The majority of maternity units have a form especially designed for this purpose. Maternity care staff should organise that the baby is clean and dressed and arrange a time for its return. It may also be a good idea to encourage the couple to take a number of photographs for their memory box.

CONCLUSION

The objective of this chapter was to compare and contrast different models of grieving and equip the reader with knowledge to critically appraise each approach. For many who experience grief, progression through psychological events is fairly straightforward and they emerge at the end of a two-year period balanced and in acceptance of what has happened to them. For a few this is not the case. For some, adjustment does not occur as quickly and/or the grieving process becomes fractured in some way. With this in mind, Chapter 5 attempts to elucidate the reader to recognise instances where a childbearing woman's grief process has become dysfunctional and when help may be required from mental health experts.

Difficulties with adjusting to the loss

In Chapter 3 we learned about the normal grief process and the classic stages of grieving according to Kubler-Ross (1969) and other models or theories that aid understanding of grief (e.g. Bowlby, 1961, 1981; Klass *et al.*, 1996; Stroebe and Schut, 1999; Worden, 1983). Grief is a normal response to loss and bereavement, and although generally the stages are the same for many people, the timing and responses may differ between individuals. For some, adjusting to the loss may become problematic, with the experiencer becoming trapped into a particular reaction that may not facilitate incorporation and adjustment to the new situation. This problematic grief may prevent the experiencer from adapting to the loss and learning to grow from the experience. Unusual responses may impact negatively on personal relationships and the ability to regain normal everyday interactions with the world. This chapter is designed to help you learn about grief that becomes challenging to the family and how to recognise instances where a childbearing woman's grief process has become maladaptive.

5.1 BEREAVEMENT AND MATERNAL MENTAL HEALTH

Maintaining mental health is important for everyone's wellbeing, but for a new mother, this is particularly the focus of the midwife. Recently, there has been a recorded rise in the number of women affected by mild to moderate mental health problems and, in some instances, psychosis during the perinatal period (Raynor and England, 2010). The impact of mental health problems experienced by childbearing women has been identified in the Confidential Enquiry into Maternal and Child Health (CEMACH) reports of 2004 and 2007 (Lewis 2004, 2007). Within these reports, maternal suicide was testimonied to be the biggest indirect cause of maternal death during the five-year period from 2000 to 2005. This finding highlights the importance of maternity care providers being vigilant about maternal mental health and developing the ability to recognise, diagnose and treat families who experience loss. The *Diagnostic and Statistical Manual of Mental Disorders* (DSM-IV-TR) (American Psychiatric Association, 2000) makes particular reference to bereavement, and specifically to its relationship to depression. It also emphasises that depression following childbirth-related bereavement differs from similar diagnosis outside childbirth (Kendler *et al.*, 2008). Despite this focused attention, the pain and impact of perinatal grief on women and their families is sometimes not acknowledged (Capitulo, 2005).

Bereavement in the perinatal period can originate from two main sources. The first source involves actual loss of a baby through miscarriage, prematurity, stillbirth or neonatal death. The second source involves loss of idealisation through events such as traumatic pregnancy or birth, producing a baby of the wrong gender, a baby that cries perpetually, having an unwell or abnormal baby, or through premature birth and loss of the cherubic infant. Enkin *et al.* (1995) and Mander (2006) discuss the colossal sense of grief that parents endure when they lose the baby they dreamed of, or their ability to engage normally in the childbearing process. Some situations can mentally traumatise the childbearing woman and leave her grieving for the experience she had fantasised about and hoped for, even when the outcome is a healthy infant.

Miscarriage adversely affects the psychological wellbeing of 50 per cent of experiencers, with symptoms persisting for up to a year post-event (Lok and Neugebauer, 2007; Séjourné *et al.*, 2010). In addition, the ordeal of pregnancy loss may result in Post Traumatic Stress Disorder and its associated unresolved grief issues (Engelhard *et al.*, 2001). The loss of a baby due to prematurity, stillbirth or neonatal death can cause serious short- and long-term distress to both parents, which may adversely affect their relationship and sabotage any opportunity for progressing to acceptance, incorporation and adaptation (Badenhorst *et al.*, 2006; Büchi *et al.*, 2008). In light of this evidence, it is important for midwives to provide care that is empathic and meets the individualised needs of childbearing women and families who are experiencing loss (Caelli *et al.*, 2002; Brier, 2008).

5.2 SIGNS AND SYMPTOMS OF DIFFICULTIES WITH ADJUSTING TO THE LOSS

A lack of a response to perinatal bereavement is considered abnormal (Capitulo, 2005), as is not adapting after a period of time to the new situation. Some responses may indicate that a woman has not progressed to accepting her new situation.

DENIAL

Although death or loss cannot be ignored indefinitely, women who remain in denial of the situation will present as coping well and do not cry in relation to their loss. Often they avoid discussions surrounding their loss and present as if life is normal. Such reactions may be due to an initial sense of shock or state of non-belief, which continues past one month post-loss.

ANGER

It is customary for the anger stage to peak at five months post-loss, with displays of wrath beyond this point considered unusual.

Displays manifest as frequent, inappropriate, unprovoked outbursts of temper directed at self and others. This is more often contained within families who disclose information to the midwife.

BARGAINING

Women stuck at a bargaining stage of grief demonstrate continued lack of acceptance. They often look for unrealistic ways to negotiate a compromise or better outcome from the situation. An example of this would be for the woman to strike a deal with God, that if she were to stop smoking, the situation would be reversed or have a better outcome.

DEPRESSION

Women who are unable to progress to acceptance, incorporation and adaptation to their loss by six months post-event may present with a symptomatic depression. During diagnosis, clinical features should not be confused with the normal feelings of sadness, regret and uncertainty that present in women who have started to accept the reality of their loss. Symptoms of depression include appetite disturbance, altered sleep patterns, lack of energy, suicidal thoughts, low mood and loss of enjoyment, anxiety, poor concentration, low self-esteem, low energy levels and loss of libido (NICE, 2007). Figure 5.1 depicts potential manifestations of grief and possible maladaptive responses at suggested points in adjustment and adaptation to the loss.

5.3 ROLE OF MATERNITY CARE PROVIDERS IN RISK ASSESSMENT

HISTORY TAKING

Good history taking has been recognised as a vital component of planning a woman's care (NICE, 2007). Of particular relevance is ensuring that care is provided by appropriate health professionals. Although it is more usual for midwives to care for women who are, by and large, well, it is also within their sphere of professional practice to make appropriate referrals and also

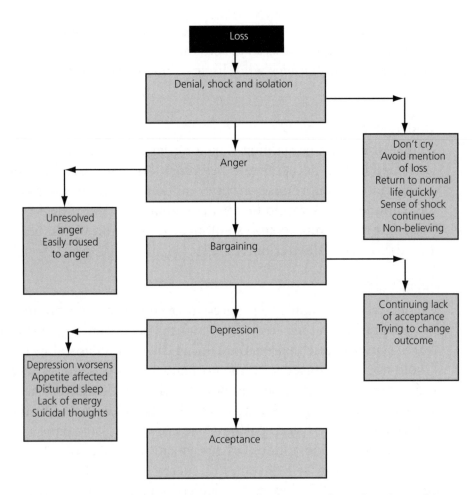

Figure 5.1 Examples of potential manifestations of grief and possible maladaptive responses at suggested points in adjustment and adaptation to loss

participate in the care of those who are sick or compromised by medical conditions. A necessary part of this role is risk assessment, which is aimed at detecting and preventing problems (NMC, 2010). Risk assessment, in part, involves taking a thorough history that includes assessment of physical, emotional and social aspects of the woman's life. Midwives are more often the first professionals to be in contact with women during the

---

Activity 11

Discuss examples where a woman does not appear to be adjusting, incorporating and adapting to her loss:

....

....

....

....

....

....

....

....

....

....

....

....

---

perinatal period. From the outset of preconception care to the end of the postnatal period, they are provided with the opportunity to develop an open and trusting therapeutic relationship with the woman (Price, 2007; Raynor and England, 2010).

Preconception visits should be arranged with women who are known to have experienced a previous loss. During the interim gap between pregnancies, ongoing support should be offered from specialists who discuss issues surrounding the loss and facilitate the woman to prepare and plan any desired future pregnancy. Specialist advice such as genetic counselling may prove beneficial. In the early stages of pregnancy, a midwife might unearth prior pregnancy loss or emotional issues affixed to a traumatic pregnancy or birth. During their interactions with women, maternity care providers are able to observe adaptive grief and identify where it becomes problematic. Appropriate responses are required if women are to be helped to untangle maladaptive aspects of grief.

Activity 12

Using the following headings, consider how you might assess a woman for signs of difficulties with adjusting, incorporating and adapting to a previous loss. Write your answers below:

Preconception advice:

....
....
....
....
....
....
....

Antenatal visits:

....
....
....
....
....
....
....
....

Postnatal visits:

....
....
....
....
....
....
....
....

Current theoretical perspectives on parental grief emphasise the importance of parents maintaining a relationship and bond with their deceased baby. Also of importance is establishing a therapeutic intervention to support parents, instead of facilitating them to minimally let go (Davies, 2004). The protocols that were examined in Chapter 1 take into account this issue. For example, Surkan *et al.* (2008) support that allowing a mother to be with her stillborn baby for as long as she wishes may positively influence symptoms of depression at a later stage. This period of bonding with the infant may assist the woman to cope better and prevent prolongation of the *depression* stage of grieving. Care providers involved in counselling grieving couples are in a position to explain the benefits of physical contact with the deceased baby in reducing the likelihood of women becoming depressed. They also require to understand that women who do not have a subsequent pregnancy are at higher risk of depression three years post loss, compared with women who became pregnant again within six months of their loss (Surkan *et al.*, 2008).

Maternity care providers need to be proactive at providing advice and offering support interventions designed to facilitate parents and families with creating meaning in their loss (Capitulo, 2008). One goal is to prevent deterioration in mental health and offset the need for referral to specialist mental health services. With this in mind, midwives should:

- provide consistent and clear advice to parents
- be compassionate in their approach to parents
- involve parents in decision-making
- provide appropriate physical and emotional support to parents
- provide relevant follow-up
- involve the multi-disciplinary team.

(Williams *et al.*, 2008)

5.4 SUBSEQUENT CARE

Unfortunately, it is not always possible to prevent mental illness. When a woman has become severely unwell during her grieving process, it is necessary to seek advice and possibly refer her to the local mental health services. For example, in Scotland there are currently two 'mother and baby' facilities. One is located in Glasgow and the other in Lothian. These units cater for women who have pre-existing mental health problems or have developed them during the perinatal period. Check out the facilities in close proximity to you. Referral to such services can be made by the midwife, health visitor or family doctor. Knowledge of specialist services and the referral protocols are important when planning ongoing care beyond the timescale of the midwife's remit. This matter will be discussed further in Chapter 5. To develop your knowledge of specialist services available in your region, complete Activity 13.

Activity 13

Find out what specialist services are available in your area for women in the perinatal period who have been bereaved and who's grieving appears to have become problematic:

....

....

....

....

....

....

....

....

....

....

....

....

....

....

....

5.5 THE MULTIDISCIPLINARY TEAM

Although midwives generally care for women in normal childbearing situations, they must recognise when the boundaries for normal processes change. As such, it is crucial for midwives to be proactive within a multidisciplinary team in order to care holistically for woman and cater for her varied needs (Midwifery, 2010). There is much evidence to support the assets of multidisciplinary team-working (NES, 2006; Reiger and Lane, 2009; Walsh and Gamble, 2005) and this is of particular relevance when providing bereavement care to women and their families. Psychiatry and, in particular, perinatal psychiatry is an obvious choice for referral of women. However, other areas of clinical expertise that could be consulted in the care of women might include clinical psychologists, fetal medicine experts, physicians and haematologists, as they all see women and families during the pre-pregnancy period to counsel and plan for future pregnancies. It might also be helpful to consider family bereavement counselling, if required. To effectively meet the needs of bereaved women who are struggling with their mental health, midwives are required to know the differing roles and responsibilities of people within the multidisciplinary team and how to access them accordingly. A co-ordinated approach to bereavement care between providers is a crucial part of ensuring that women and families receive appropriate and vital support (Scottish Government, 2011).

5.6 WHEN GRIEF BECOMES PROBLEMATIC

At this point in the workbook the reader should be able to identify causes and manifestations of problematic grief. Equipped with this information, read the scenarios in Activities 14, 15, and 16 and answer the questions asked. Respectively, consider what actions of care planning each woman in the individual case study requires.

> *Note:*
> Remember to consider each woman and her situation as unique. Women respond to grief in many different ways.

Activity 14

List the key professions involved in the care of bereaved women:

....

....

....

....

....

....

Discuss how you would access each profession:

....

....

....

....

....

....

....

....

....

....

....

5.7 GRIEF AND LATE TERMINATION FOR FETAL ABNORMITY

During pregnancy, childbearing women are offered a range of
tests, scans and screening procedures that offer information about
progress of the developing fetus. Although screening provides
reassurance for the majority of childbearing couples, some will be
told that their baby may have a serious abnormality. Upon
confirmation of abnormality, the woman will be asked how she
wants her pregnancy to proceed. For a choice about termination
of pregnancy to be afforded, within UK law the fetus will be
required to be under 24 weeks' gestational age. In England,
Scotland and Wales, the Abortion Act (1967) specifies that

Activity 15

Petra is 34 years old and has been trying for a baby for five years. She has just experienced her sixth miscarriage. You are the maternity care professional involved in Petra's pregnancy and did not know her before this event. When you visit Petra at home for a postnatal follow-up, she tells you that she is returning to work the next day.

What issues might be affecting Petra at this time?

....
....
....
....
....

How would you recognise if Petra was adjusting to her loss?

....
....
....
....
....

What advice would you give to Petra and why?

....
....
....
....
....
....

What follow-up do you arrange for Petra and why?

....
....
....
....

Activity 16

Roseanne has four healthy boys. She is now 32 weeks' gestation and in her fifth pregnancy. She attends for a routine antenatal check-up and tells you that she has been having recurring dreams in which she sees that the baby is a boy. She admits to feeling distressed by this occurrence and states that her emotions and thoughts are affecting her mood and appetite.

Although this pregnancy is progressing well, what features indicate that Roseanne could be experiencing a grief reaction in this situation?

....

....

....

....

....

What advice would you give to Roseanne and why?

....

....

....

....

....

....

....

What follow-up care plan would you discuss with Roseanne?

....

....

....

....

....

....

....

....

Activity 17

Saliha is a 30-year-old woman who was 32 weeks' gestation and in her third pregnancy when she had endured an antepartum haemorrhage. The cause of the haemorrhage was disruption of a type three placenta praevia. During preparation for an emergency caesarean section, it was discovered that there was an absent fetal heartbeat. Following the birth of her dead baby daughter, Saliha made a good physical recovery and displayed normal grieving symptoms. Six months later, both Saliha and her husband attend a pre-pregnancy counselling session, because they desire to conceive another baby. At this meeting Saliha's husband mentions that she goes into the nursery every day to search for her baby and still talks in disbelief and shock that she is not there. Her husband affirms that he finds this circumstance a challenge to manage.

How would you respond to this situation?

....
....
....
....
....

What indicators make you think that Saliha has not adjusted, incorporated or adapted to her loss?

....
....
....
....

What follow-up care plan would you discuss with Saliha and her husband?

....
....
....
....

termination of pregnancy beyond 24 weeks of gestation is only legal if either the fetus is at substantial risk of serious handicap or there is a risk of grave permanent injury to the life, or the physical or mental health, of the childbearing woman. Once the 'bad news' has been broken the childbearing woman will require time to discuss matters with her family and consider the best course of action for her personal circumstances. In some instances, early delivery may be necessary to protect the health of the pregnant woman, either because of intense bleeding, possible development of complications during pregnancy, which may threaten her life, or because the fetus is at risk *in utero*. The most common complications are maternal pre-eclampsia, which place both parties at risk. In particular, the fetus is at risk of developing Intrauterine Growth Retardation (IUGR) and/or *fetal distress* through restriction of blood supply to the placenta. The sense of balance between risk to the fetus of remaining in the uterus, against risk of death and disability after premature delivery, requires to be assessed carefully.

In the UK, protocols for screening for fetal abnormality are routinely offered during pregnancy. These include screening for Down's syndrome and fetal anomalies such as hydrocephalus, limb abnormalities, haemoglobinopathies and rhesus haemolytic disease. For fetal chromosome abnormalities, screening is conducted through ultrasound measurement of the nuchal translucency between 10 and 14 weeks' gestation and/or maternal blood analysis at 10–20 weeks of pregnancy.

Late termination will inevitably traumatise the childbearing woman, partner, relatives and friends, as she is perhaps ending a profoundly wanted pregnancy, and, in particular, when she is required to labour and give birth. If above 22 weeks' gestation, her fetus may show signs of life at delivery, such as a heartbeat, gasp or reflex movements. The birth of a live child in such a case requires to be registered, which parents and staff may find distressing, in particular following termination.

The Royal College of Obstetricians and Gynaecologists (RCOG) (2001a) have developed guidelines that include the recommendation that feticide (causing the death of a fetus) be carried out before the initiation of labour in terminations after 21 weeks and six days' gestation, to ensure that the fetus is not born alive. The recommended method of feticide is an injection of potassium chloride into the fetal heart (RCOG, 2001b), which halts the fetal heartbeat. It is mostly regarded as a means of causing rapid death and does not require analgesia. Feticide pre-empts the possibility of dilemmas surrounding whether a baby born alive after termination should be resuscitated. Some parents have reported relief at knowing their baby will not suffer during induced labour or be born alive, and others report experiencing distress (Statham *et al.*, 2001). Interview studies with parents have found that when the procedure is handled sensitively, reactions to feticide appear not to dominate the experience of grief at the loss of a wanted baby. In 2005, 31 per cent (approximately 800) of the terminations that took place at 20 weeks' gestation onwards in England and Wales were reported to include feticide (Government Statistical Service, 2006). What is important is that staff should feel able to respect the woman's wish if she chooses to decline feticide. In these circumstances, thorough discussions with the woman and her partner about the likely outcomes should take place. It is important that the childbearing woman should be given time to consider her decision and evaluate whether termination without feticide genuinely is what she wants. If so, she should agree a care plan in advance of the procedure that covers possible outcomes.

Discussions should surround effects of the abnormality upon the child, upon themselves and upon other immediate family members (including children they may have in the future). In addition, it is important to discuss prior attitudes and beliefs surrounding termination of pregnancy. When making such harrowing decisions, it has been suggested that parents tend not to focus on levels of risk and the available options in an objective way, but rather on their perceptions of self-coping (Statham, 2002).

LEGAL STATUS OF THE FATHER

At a legal level, a childbearing woman does not have to take into account the wishes of the baby's father. Whilst the requirements of the law are clear, carers should ensure that the childbearing woman is able to make an informed choice about her pregnancy and its outcomes. This requires effective communication skills to help her understand associated risks to herself and fetus and any subsequent pregnancies. If the fetal complication is hereditary, it is important that she meets with a genetic counsellor to ascertain risk of conceiving a fetus with the same chromosomal disorder.

PROFESSIONAL RESPONSIBILITY

When a member of staff has a conscientious objection to termination of pregnancy, they have the right under the Abortion Act (1967) to refuse to participate in such procedures. This right of conscientious objection towards participating in the termination is supported by the Royal College of Midwives (RCM) and the British Medical Association (BMA). There is however a moral obligation not to influence the woman's decision to have feticide or termination. Dilemmas that relate should be considered when designating a member of staff to liaise with and provide care to the woman and her partner. It should also be considered that modern medicine can augment distress. For example, medical imaging that visualises the fetus in three dimensions and depicts movements inside the uterus can augment parental distress and influence their decision-making.

CONCLUSION

The objective of this chapter is to teach the reader to recognise when a woman's grief process has become problematic and how and where to seek help when the event occurs. Upon recovery, the couple may wish to seek information about what they can achieve in the future, e.g. when it is safe for them to become pregnant again after a perinatal loss and the incumbent risks that may be involved. Presently, there is no evidence about the best time to attempt to conceive another baby after a stillbirth. Ultimately, the

CASE STUDY

Candy is a single 19-year-old woman with an unplanned first pregnancy. She discovered that she was pregnant at 23 weeks and, once adjusted to the idea, was happy. After a series of tests, it was discovered that the fetus had severe spinabifida. In this condition, some areas of the spine fail to develop, often resulting in spastic paralysis. A scan at 18 weeks' gestation revealed the problem. Candy was offered the option of terminating her pregnancy because the prospects for the fetus were so severe. If born alive, the child would have severe disability and be unable to walk. Candy was very upset because she no longer was carrying the baby she hoped for. Candy was offered feticide as stage one of the termination procedure. She agreed to termination, but was unsure about the idea of feticide because the responsibility for agreeing to the euthanasia of her infant caused her distress.

Making the decision to end the pregnancy

Those who hold that there is a moral obligation to preserve life at all costs would not sanction termination or the foregoing feticide. Others might think that there would be minimal advantages to the baby being born alive, and maintain that to preserve life was cruel.

Consider the following points:

- Candy may or may not hold definite views about the rightness or wrongness of termination and/or feticide.
- Whatever Candy decides, this is likely to be a disturbing experience.
- Candy may perceive pressure from staff towards a particular decision.
- Candy may feel guilt at the prospect of agreeing to terminate her pregnancy.
- Candy may feel that she is responsible for causing the spinabifida.
- Candy may feel she needs a lot of counselling. Psychological and spiritual assistance may be of value to her. Why?
- Were Candy to agree to feticide, she will have to cope with taking responsibility for the death of her baby.
- Candy's relatives may have very different views to her about the situation, which may cause concern if she derives her sense of morality from their attitudes. She may also be influenced by those who hold strong religious or disability rights perspectives.

decision is the couple's. They may, however, want to talk events through with a midwife, obstetrician, geneticist, counsellor or hospital chaplain. Understandably, becoming pregnant again may be anxiety-provoking and a time to seek counselling about fears.

Chapter 6 concerns itself with outlining the processes that are available to provide support of many varieties of loss post-discharge from the maternity unit. For example, associations like the Stillbirth and Neonatal Death Society (SANDS) have produced many helpful booklets, and the National Childbirth Trust (NCT) have a shared experiences helpline.

6

Ongoing support

Learning objective addressed

On completion of Chapter 6 the reader should be able to:

6. Outline processes involved in caring for and advising a bereaved woman/partner/family about how to access ongoing support on discharge from maternity care.

Having previously discussed how to recognise when a woman's grief process has become problematical, it is important to be aware of referral pathways for women and their families. Chapter 5 has been designed to inform you about the processes involved in caring for and advising a bereaved woman and her family about how to access ongoing support on discharge from midwifery care.

6.1 ROLE OF PROFESSIONALS IN BEREAVEMENT CARE

Grief following the loss of a child is recognised to be one of the most intense and difficult categories of loss to tackle. Associated bereavement impacts on the entire family and social structure and therefore poses a challenge to care providers. During the antenatal period, parents psychologically prepare for a life incorporating the unborn child, which involves development of attachments that continue following birth (Condon, 2010). When the baby dies, loss of the potential relationship can create a discordant grieving cycle associated with a myriad of feelings, one of which is anxiety. In Rosemary Mander's (2006) book *Loss and Bereavement in Childbearing*, she discusses how Bowlby (1990) viewed grief as an adult version of child separation anxiety that manifests with similar feelings.

Midwives and allied health and social care professionals are in an ideal position to support women during pregnancy, childbirth and the puerperium (O'Lunaigh and Carlson, 2005). As part of this role, they require to provide appropriate tailor-made support and education to women experiencing perinatal bereavement (Williams *et al.*, 2008). Professionals who provide compassionate personalised care to the woman are more effective at relieving grief and promoting a normal bereavement process. Within this role, in order to provide effective care, it is essential for carers to be aware of their own feelings about bereavement. A carer who feels uncomfortable may act impersonally, assume a superior role and/or make decisions for the parents (Capitulo, 2005). Consequently, it is important for them to reflect on their own feelings about handling bereavement and consider whether they can provide an open and empathic response during support provision to a bereaved woman and her family. More specifically, carers can facilitate certain practical functions that promote a healing response for parents' grief. Some interventions that require inclusion follow:

GOOD COMMUNICATION

Good communication includes allowing the parents to talk and tell their story of pregnancy, birth and loss, and provide some validity to their bereavement by using helpful expressions such as 'I understand your baby has died' and 'I'm so sorry about that'. The use of the word 'died' helps to convey the reality of the situation and should be used rather than saying 'passed away'. Also, statements such as 'You're young and can always have another baby' should be avoided.

SUPPORT FOR LOSS

Although maternity professionals work with women in the first 10–14 days after birth, this period can be extended in particular circumstances. To provide adaptable care, these professional carers need to have a clear understanding of the different types of loss that women and families can experience. The type of loss may be transparent, as occurs when a woman has a miscarriage, stillbirth or neonatal death. Conversely, it may not be so obvious, as when a woman's expectations are dashed by a traumatic birth, unwanted gender of baby or ill neonate. Once a loss has been recognised, it is necessary to action appropriate care. Type of support required by an individual woman is dependent upon how she frames her loss and the type of loss experienced. An inventory of types of support and services follows:

Early pregnancy loss/miscarriage
- Consent for investigation of fetus
- Obstetrician consultation
- Between pregnancy testing
- Pre-pregnancy counselling
- Genetics counselling
- Contraceptive advice
- Multidisciplinary notification
- Specialist appointments

Stillbirth/neonatal death
- Memory moments
- Cultural sensitivity
- Post mortem
- Undertaker
- Obstetrician/paediatrician consultation
- Bereavement counselling
- Multidisciplinary notification

Loss of expectations
- Pregnancy and birth debriefing
- Counselling services
- Pre-pregnancy counselling
- Multidisciplinary notification
- Pregnancy care plan

6.2 GENDER AND ETHNICITY AND THE IMPORTANCE OF NOT STEREOTYPING

Gender and ethnicity can shape individual experiences of bereavement. The timing, place, manner and social implications of a person's death are shaped by their age, ethnicity, gender, social class and sexuality. All of these factors influence ways people experience death, dying and bereavement. Such forms of social differentiation are produced through the approaches we have towards living our lives. The ways in which a particular society manages death reveals much about their value systems. Notably, burial traditions demonstrate the magnitude to which people are valued within their society.

There is a significant number of differences in mortality and illness between men and women in the UK and other western societies, with doctors and nurses responding differentially to clients along gender lines. For example, more women are diagnosed as having mental health problems, whilst men are more likely to require heart surgery. Another difference relates to biological factors that link with susceptibility to death and disease. For example, genetic factors are linked with higher rates of miscarriage and infant mortality in male babies, whilst women are more likely to develop breast cancer. Differing hormone profiles between the sexes are considered to be linked to various medical conditions.

Several researchers argue that gender differences in death and illness are the product of differing patterns of behaviour and lifestyles between men and women. In other words, differences are connected to gender roles within society. Help-seeking and emotionality are ingredients of conventional ideas about female roles, whereas males are expected to confine expression of emotion, refute illness and demonstrate reluctance to ask for help. As a consequence, help-seeking and giving can become harmonised with romanticised female gender roles in western society.

The attitudes of maternity care staff may contribute to the difficulties some parents experience in handling guilt. In pre-industrial societies there were high death rates at the beginning of life, and as such, young life was less highly valued. Entry to society was marked through survival, when a naming ceremony took place. At this point the baby became socially acknowledged as a member of the community. Deaths before this time were barely recognised and neonatal deaths and stillbirths did not receive full funeral rites (Hertz, 1960).

The grief of women whose babies have died *in utero*, are stillborn or have been neonatal deaths is made legitimate through bureaucratic and ritual procedures that legitimise the baby as an individual with a social identity. There are gendered responses to grief in the ways fathers and mothers try to make sense of the death of their baby. Bowlby (1981) drew on studies of grieving widows for the purpose of developing models of bereavement that systematise bereavement into a universal process, as opposed to a culturally developed experience. As a consequence, whilst a generic model is taken as equally applicable to both men and women, these theories, in the main, reflect experiences of married women. Practically, there are important differences between men and women in relation to how they approach death.

Gender differences in patterns of bereavement care prevail, with female relatives providing the bulk of the emotional care to those who are grieving. In addition, where the husband is the main carer, he is more likely to receive support. Experiences of death are conceptualised in the ways carers are trained. Emphasis is placed on meeting the needs of grieving individuals in a holistic way. Cultural and behavioural differences are prevalent explanations for ethnic inequalities in health. Minority ethnic communities in the UK may maintain distinctive definitions of illness and traditions of healthcare and, as such, knowledge of and attitudes towards health and social care services may affect use. As such, definitions of symptoms and relating to healthcare professionals vary between cultures and ethnic minorities. Language difficulties, religious differences and family customs may generate or exacerbate misunderstandings between minority group members and their carers.

It is important not to be ethnocentric and insensitive to cultural differences. Such action may symbolise a service that represents a specific pattern of thinking. For example, taking the isolated nuclear family as the norm may lead to ignoring and excluding extended family from participating in the birth of a stillborn infant or neonate. Ethnic differences and religious customs must be considered during physical procedures, such as rituals surrounding visiting and managing a sick neonate, preferred diet and dealings with death and dying. Recognition of such factors has led to the view that health workers need to be aware of and show respect for the values, beliefs and traditions of minority ethnic patients.

On occasion, attempts to use a cultural approach may be unrealistic, particularly when intended to alter a lifestyle. As such, they could be interpreted as being demeaning and inadvertently racist. Respect for class inequalities during delivery of bereavement care are less often acknowledged in discussions about deprived minority ethnic communities. For example, one factor identified is that unemployment is greater in the majority of minority ethnic groups. Racism and discrimination have significant, although difficult to specify, influences upon perinatal death management. The lifestyles of people from another culture are sometimes portrayed as being illogical, outlandish and less significant. The implication of this is that minority communities should resolve differences by embracing more sensible western ways. It is important that health and social care professionals are respectful of all people, with neglect to do so sometimes resulting in client failure to attend for vital clinic appointments, and as such this produces lowered service utilisation.

Ethnicity, like gender, is an important source of social identity, which must be acknowledged and respected by health and social care professionals who work with grieving couples who have experienced, or are about to experience, a perinatal death. It is important to recognise that each person, be they health professional, volunteer, patient or family member, has their own unique understanding of life and its meaning. For example, within one western nuclear family there may be one member who is atheist, whilst the others are agnostic, Buddhist, Christian, Muslim, Hindu or Spiritualist. Differences in one social group have been moulded by ethnic origins, social class, family expectations, prior exposure to religion and philosophy.

To operate as an effective member of the helping professions, one must first understand themselves in relation to their own social customs, prejudices and world view. It is important to work out one's own structure and meaning. Through full awareness of our own beliefs, we can develop empathy and cultural sensitivity to the values and needs of others. One method of doing this would be to develop a 'death plan' for ourselves in which we plan how we would like to die and the funeral we would like to have. This process bears similarity to writing a birth plan (Hollins Martin, 2008). Writing an 'end of life plan' with the childbearing couple would help the carer construct individual meaning and clear up any complications of ambiguity about cultural differences. In other words, providing the family with choice and control is important.

CONCEPTUALISING THE RELATIONSHIP BETWEEN PERINATAL DEATH, GENDER AND ETHNICITY

There is a multitude of effects that can result from demographic factors. For example:

- a persons expectations of life
- a person's desire for relocation
- the amount of money a person is expected to have
- the number and value of material items a person owns
- expectations of family members and what constitutes success in their eyes
- acceptable gender relationships
- expectations of healthcare
- secularisation and effects upon patterns of death, dying and bereavement
- urbanisation and effects upon patterns of death, dying and bereavement.

In essence, relationships between individuals and groups within the broader social structure and shape influence their lives. Any adequate account of relationships between death, gender and ethnicity must be informed by a view of the nature of a person's society. The theoretical assumption behind this landscape is that societies and organisations have a social reality of their own, regardless of the individuals of which they consist. When delivering perinatal bereavement care, those concerned must acknowledge the complexities that lie hidden underneath the individual childbearing women's desires for the loss she is coming to terms with, and that of her partner, which may considerably differ. It is important to remember that families consist of different but interrelated parts, which coexist in some sort of stable balance. Thus change in one part of the family, for example loss of an infant, will have consequences for other aspects of the family and its structure. In differing circumstances, loss of a perinate may affect parental separation rates and/or increase the chance of developing a stress-related illness.

Differences in the health of minority ethnic groups result from their economic position within society. Most women and most minority ethnic groups are economically disadvantaged within capitalist societies. They are also politically and socially disadvantaged and, as a result, females often have inferior health than more advantaged males and the dominant ethnic group. Whilst gender and ethnicity are themselves important social divisions, they are not homogeneous but, instead, heterogeneous groupings. These views influence the relationship between beliefs and practices by which perinatal death is managed. The point made herein is that emphasis also needs to be given to death and dying within its wider social context through asking what death rituals reveal about the broader structuring of social life; for example, how female and male infants are viewed and how the deceased infant is managed. The following case is designed to emphasise cultural differences in the way gender is viewed.

The emphasis of the aforementioned case study is upon enlightening that there are multifaceted structures that provide

CASE STUDY

Primrose is a 29-year-old first-generation Chinese lady who is having a planned first pregnancy. She and her husband (Nelson) are on a one-year trip to the UK to set up a business liaison for the Chinese company in which Nelson is employed. Primrose is 17 weeks' pregnant and has just had her first scan, which revealed that their baby is female. On all measures the baby appears healthy and is developing appropriately. Both Primrose and her husband perceive that they need a boy, because culture within Chinese society dictates that sons are responsible for looking after their parents in their old age. It is a daughter's responsibility to care for her husband's parents. Also, the Chinese state they live in operates a single-child policy for every couple. Nelson asks how much it will cost to have a termination of pregnancy. Primrose agrees that she also wants a termination, but is unsure how she will cope.

Consider the following points:

■ What is Primrose and Nelson's legal standing within the UK in relation to their request for termination?
■ What is Primrose and Nelson's legal standing within China in relation to their request for termination?
■ Primrose may or may not hold definite views about the rightness or wrongness of this termination.
■ Whatever Primrose decides, this is likely to be a disturbing experience for them both.
■ Primrose may perceive pressure from Nelson towards their decision to have a termination for gender reasons.
■ Nelson may perceive pressure from his wife towards their decision to have a termination for gender reasons.
■ One or both parents may feel guilt at the prospect of agreeing to terminate their pregnancy.
■ Primrose may feel she is responsible for the situation.
■ Primrose and/or Nelson may feel they need counselling. Would psychological and spiritual assistance within the UK system be of value to them and why?
■ Were Primrose to agree to the termination, she will have to cope with the death of her baby.

■ Relatives, who are thousands of miles away may have very different views to both Primrose and Nelson.

■ As the health, social or pastoral care professional involved in this case, what are your own thoughts and emotions about the request for termination of pregnancy and should they be used to persuade a decision?

coherence to the management of both life and death of this particular fetus. The case study does not fully address either the range of meanings and functions or values that the couple operate with. Nonetheless, the case study offers a fruitful approach to theorising gender and ethnicity based differences between two societies. Specifically, this case emphasises the roles of individuals in shaping and controlling behaviour. Particular emphasis is placed upon communication between carer and couple in relation to perceived crises along the way and management of the dilemma and negotiation about what values are acceptable and transferable between individual societies.

Also of relevance, is how the social organisation of maternity units constrain and shape what is acceptable or unacceptable within their remit. For example, termination on grounds of sex alone currently is not permitted in UK society, but acceptable in China. As such, this case study addresses the broader effect of social constraints upon individuals from political structures. Although valuable at the individual level, they can make only a limited contribution to our understanding of broader social factors. The case study also explains reactions to gender and worth within the experiencing of individual rather than social contexts and social relationships within which these experiences occur. The ethnocentric framework raises questions about behaviour of females and males from two differing cultures. In addition, misgivings and misunderstandings of midwives, doctors, radiographers, nurses, social workers, spiritual carers, counsellors and other professionals cannot be undervalued. Understanding and accepting relationships between gender and death and between ethnicity and death are an ongoing challenge for such professionals.

6.3 SUPPORT SERVICES

SUPPORT GROUPS

Health and social care professionals can advise parents of additional help available from support groups. Although these might not be suitable for all women, professionals can provide information about them and let the woman make her own judgements. Research suggests that support groups are particularly helpful to those parents who are able to create meaningful memories of their baby (Côté-Arsenault and Morrison-Beedy, 2001; Calhoun *et al.*, 2003; Capitulo, 2005). Consequently, it is important for the maternity care providers to promote positive memories. In addition, there are numerous voluntary organisations who offer specialised support to women who are experiencing bereavement. Care providers should provide women and their families with details about how to contact these organisations. Examples follow:

CRUSE

www.crusebereavementcare.org.uk
Telephone: 0844 477 9400
Cruse is an organisation that attempts to facilitate the bereaved person to understand their grief and cope with their loss. As well as providing free care to all bereaved people, the charity also offers information, support and training services to those who are looking after bereaved persons. Cruse is a member of the British Association of Counsellors and Psychotherapists and follows the rigorous code of ethics set out by that organisation. The welfare services that Cruse provides, particularly via its telephone helpline, have also been awarded a Quality Mark by Community Legal Advice.

Derby Hospitals NHS Foundation Trust
Library and Knowledge Service

SANDS
www.uk-sands.org
Telephone: 020 7436 5881
The Stillbirth and Neonatal Death Society (SANDS) is an organisation that can offer support to the woman and her family when their baby dies during pregnancy or after birth. The death of a baby is a devastating experience and effects of grief can be overwhelming to parents, their families and friends who can be left feeling dazed, disorientated, isolated and exhausted. At SANDS, members of the organisation have often been through the experience and therefore can identify with what the woman is experiencing, and offer support and information where needed. For example, when a baby has been stillborn or has died during or soon after birth, or has spent some time in a special care baby unit (SCBU). It may be that the baby died at an earlier gestation or that a difficult decision to end the pregnancy was required. SANDS offer support to mothers, fathers and other members of the family, including grandparents and other siblings.

BLISS
www.bliss.org.uk
Telephone: 0500 618140
Bliss exists to ensure that all babies born too soon, too small or too sick in the UK have the best possible chance of survival and of reaching their full potential. Members of Bliss support mothers and families of babies that are premature, making sure that the voices of babies and families are heard. By driving quality and innovation in the NHS, Bliss works to improve care provision for premature and sick babies and their families.

THE MISCARRIAGE ASSOCIATION
www.miscarriageassociation.org.uk
Helpline: 01924 200799
The Miscarriage Association acknowledges the distress associated with pregnancy loss and strives to make a positive difference to those it affects, including the father and other children. It aims to:

- offer support and information to anyone affected by the loss of a baby in pregnancy
- raise awareness of miscarriage
- promote good practice in medical care.

SAMARITANS
www.samaritans.org
Telephone: 08457 909090
Samaritans provide a confidential emotional support service to residents of the United Kingdom and Ireland who are experiencing distress, despair or suicidal feelings. Support is available 24 hours a day. The service is staffed by volunteers who respond to phone calls, emails and letters. Alternatively, members of the community can visit a branch of the Samaritans, where they can have a face-to-face meeting with an affiliate of the organisation.

THE FAMILY BEREAVEMENT COUNSELLING SERVICE
http://www.nhsggc.org.uk
Telephone: 0141 201 9257
The Family Bereavement Counselling Service at Yorkhill Hospital offers bereavement and counselling support for users and staff of GG&C Health Board. Anyone affected by miscarriage, stillbirth or termination can be offered one-to-one support, telephone support and befriending services. A lending library is also available for use. Although a local service to a specific region in Scotland, there are many localised services in the different cities of the UK.

6.4 GRIEF COUNSELLING
Losing a born or unborn infant can be a very disappointing and lonely experience. Amongst family and friends it can be very testing for the couple to explain the details, particularly if they did not actually know the woman was childbearing. As such, circumstances will potentially restrain how events will unfold and assessment of support that may be needed. In essence, others may not grasp the full extent of the loss actually experienced by the childbearing

---

Activity 18

There are many recognised organisations that provide support to grieving parents and families. Identify what additional support is available in your local community and list these below:

....

....

....

....

....

....

....

Provide the contact details of these additional organisations:

....

....

....

....

....

---

woman, partner, family and close friends. Some people may fail to recognise that the couple may have lost their dreams and hopes for their future and, as such, phrases to avoid include:

'Never mind, you'll get pregnant again soon.'
'Oh well, it was only a miscarriage.'
'It is probably for the best; perhaps something was wrong with the baby.'

The extent of the tragedy can only be acknowledged by each member of the couple on an individual basis, with differences in thoughts and response behaviours often differing between the two of them. Every individual measures and deals with loss in their own unique style. Social values and circumstances vary between personalities, cultures and families and as such will direct the extent and depth of a person's grief process. During conversations with the childbearing woman and her partner it is important to discuss the following:

- Stages of the grief process and common symptoms that may be experienced. Commonplace symptoms of grief include:
  - crying
  - feelings of hopelessness
  - feelings of helplessness
  - self-blame
  - guilt
  - sleep disturbances
  - appetite disturbance
  - irritability
  - anger
  - forgetfulness
  - feeling emotionally numb
  - feeling empty
  - feeling lonely
  - feeling isolated
  - recurring desire to talk about death and related events
  - disorderliness in everyday life
  - despairing about future and what it will bring
  - lack of concentration
  - problems with planning future goals
  - difficulties with remembering information.

- Encounters of grief can affect a person's perceptions of the world. For example, after experiencing hurt and healing the world will return to a different 'normal'.
- There is no timetable of the grief process to follow. Events and time taken to progress through the stages of grief will differ between members of the family. Individuals take varying amounts of time to feel the emotions of each stage and the order may vary. Some steps may go completely amiss. Explain possible stages of grief that may be experienced:

- shock and denial
- anger and guilt
- depression and loneliness
- acceptance and hope.

- It is entirely usual for grieving styles and experiences to differ between both members of the couple.
- Sharing experiences of loss and thoughts with others who offer to listen may bring a great deal of comfort and strong feelings of connectedness.
- Many couples find solace in support groups and/or counsellors. Provide information about how to access various forms of support. Explain that the offer may be taken up at any point in the process and that what is selected may not suit both members of the couple. Some like to talk to others who have had similar losses, whilst others favour support from a psychotherapist or professional counsellor. The couple may elect to see a therapist together.
- It is important to seek help from a professional who has experience in grief counselling related to perinatal loss. This is a highly unique situation that requires sophisticated understanding of the childbearing cycle, as well as knowledge of the specific medical interventions or illnesses that surround the loss.
- There may be difficult encounters during the grieving process. For example:
  - meeting friends and family with new babies
  - seeing people with new babies in prams
  - baby showers and religious rites of passage, e.g. christenings or equivalent baby welcoming or naming ceremonies
  - encounters with breastfeeding mothers
  - dealing with unhelpful comments, e.g. 'When are you planning to try again?'
  - returning to the maternity unit for check-ups.

- Provide some pain-easing tips:
  - Select your confidants carefully. Avoid those you know are ill-equipped to manage or simply just do not have the skills required for healthy discussion.
  - Be forthright with people who upset you. Just say thank you and that you do not want to talk about it.
  - Find a source of support outside your partner. A couple may exhaust each other with their discussions and may be at differing points in the grieving process.
  - Make time to spend with your partner. Put appointments in your diary for each other.
  - Eat, rest, exercise and take care of yourself.
  - If you cannot face children's parties, baby showers and naming ceremonies, be polite and give your apologies.
  - Avoid making major decisions until you feel in balance again.
  - Be patient with your partner. They may be very different to you in how they handle feelings, events and people.
  - Remember you always have the numbers of support groups you can contact.
  - Keep a memory box of items connected with the baby or pregnancy, e.g. ultrasound photographs, hospital records, a lock of hair etc.
  - Consider attending a counselling group. It may be helpful to share experiences with others who have had similar experiences of loss.
  - Be good to yourself. Enjoy treats, e.g. buy flowers you like, chocolates, have a warm bath etc. You deserve them.

It is really important that the couple can recognise when their grief process is taking a wrong turn. Advise them to seek help when their grief turns to despair and begins to affect their daily coping and living skills. They must be taught to recognise this point in each other. Explain that grieving can be hard work and quite fatiguing. Fortitude is required to obtain the point of remedy. Advise that with time, healing will occur and that they will reach a point where they have integrated their experience of loss into their life and can coexist with it comfortably. From their experience of loss they will grow and learn skills to deal with further similar situations and gain understanding and empathy for others experiencing similar events. In fact, many counsellors have been drawn to their role through experiences of emotional difficulties that relate to the baby blues, pregnancy, the postpartum period, miscarriage, pregnancy loss, infant loss, infertility and adoption etc.

WHAT ARE THE OBJECTIVES OF GRIEF COUNSELLING?

Fundamentally, grief counselling facilitates people who are grieving to get their lives back on track. The following objectives are involved:

1. *Listening* – It is of key importance to listen to what the grieving individual has to say. Attempts to understand the context in which their feelings are embedded may require the counsellor to ask a few questions. Having someone who listens carefully may help them to progress through their grief process. This, in fact, may be all that is required, since in many cases grief may not be a particularly challenging emotion for which the couple requires support. In many cases the childbearing woman's friends and family members may find it difficult to provide the support that is needed because they are also grieving. Grief counselling allows that person to talk about how they feel without constraint and fear of upsetting another who is experiencing the same loss.

2. *Refocusing* – After a perinatal death it may be difficult for a person to get their life back on track. For a while they may become unstable, insecure and disinclined to return to work. Counselling may help the individual construct a recovery calendar that gently levers them back into their more standard routine world. A constructive counsellor will attempt to pull the griever back from a descending spiral by spotlighting healthy and happy events in their life and drawing them back from negative thought processes.

3. *Routine* – If the childbearing woman and partner commit to a series of grief counselling sessions, it must be pointed out to them that they will be following a schedule that may address different aspects of their grieving at each attendance. Consequently, it is a good idea to attend each session and not miss any. Whilst the woman may find returning to her pre-pregnancy life daunting, attending the grief counsellor may form one steady routine in a week. Through attendance she will leave her house and face the world outside her front door.

4. *Managing complicated emotions* – Everybody grieves differently and yet often with similarity. The subtle variations can be discussed with a grief counsellor. For example, some people lash out at those around them and become destructive. Some can develop physical ailments. Some experience no pain whatsoever and are finally assaulted by it months later. In relation to the array of individual responses, grief counselling can help people with complicated emotions cope more effectively. Through discussion, their thoughts and feelings can be worked through in a safe environment in which others are not exposed to hurtful assaults.

The psychology of counselling is a specialty that embraces research and applied disciplines in numerous extensive domains. To train to become a counsellor involves extensive training and supervision and there are several approaches; for example, cognitive behavioral therapy (CBT), person-centered counselling, mindfulness and psychotherapy. There are professional journals that publish research in the area of counselling; for example:

- *The Journal of Counseling Psychology*
- *The Counseling Psychologist*
- *The European Journal of Counselling Psychology*
- *Counselling Psychology Quarterly.*

To be accredited as a counsellor, one must have completed an accredited programme, some of which are at graduate, Master's and PhD level.

A CASE STUDY OF VERY SPECIFIC CULTURAL CONSIDERATIONS IN BEREAVEMENT CARE

Pavlish (2005) obtained narrative data from Congolese refugee women. Through analysis of discussions the extent of atrocities experienced became apparent. Grieving was prolonged for some, due to severity of loss to their lives and a resigned belief that, culturally, many aspects of their life could not be changed. Many African cultures have a patriarchal system, with men in the dominant role and women submissive. Such societal organisation may contribute to the ways women respond when faced with loss and bereavement. Read the following scenario based on an anonymous factual event and consider the woman's situation and reaction to the news she has received. Analyse your perceptions of how you think this young woman should be reacting.

CASE STUDY

Rosette was tortured, raped and has witnessed the brutal murder of her mother by soldiers in her village in the war-torn area of the Congo. Rosette has arrived in the UK where she has been granted asylum. Upon arrival she was found to be around seven months' pregnant and a blood test has diagnosed her as HIV positive. You are the maternity care professional assigned to care for her. During the process of conducting an ultrasonic scan you are unable to detect the fetal heartbeat or identify fetal movements. Rosette does not wish to speak about what has happened to her and tells the interpreter that she has given this problem to Jesus. She states that God is the only one who cares for her.

Consider the following points:

- What factors within this scenario arouse your concern?
- How would you manage the individual problems that you have identified?
- How would you manage Rosette's HIV positive status?
- Rosette may benefit from counselling. What psychological and spiritual assistance within the system would be of value to her and why?

Write a care plan that addresses Rosette's unique and specific needs.

CONCLUSION

The objective of this chapter is to outline processes involved in caring for and advising a bereaved woman/partner and family about how to access ongoing support on discharge from the maternity unit. Losing a pregnancy or infant can be a very disappointing experience for the couple. Similarly, it can be an upsetting event for the professionals and ancillary staff who become involved. It is important to recognise that they too may have had personal experience of perinatal bereavement that becomes activated by the event. They may also have lost their dreams and hopes in a similar way, or feel they are responsible for the events that have unfolded. Such staff responses must be acknowledged and considered acceptable. Remember midwives are not robots who perform in an emotionless way when confronted with sentiment-filled events. What they must do is recognise their own dilemma and ask to leave the situation. As in all dealings, another may be better equipped to handle this particular set of circumstances. Empathy is rooted in emotional intelligence, which is underpinned by the ability to experience and express emotion.

In essence, Chapter 7 concerns itself with outlining how colleagues can recognise when a bereavement incident has stressed a peer member of staff and how to remedy the situation. The motto espoused is that 'colleagues must provide peer support to one another'.

7

Staff support

Learning objective addressed

On completion of Chapter 7 the reader should be able to:

7. Recognise where a bereavement incident may affect a member of staff adversely.

For the most part, there are positive outcomes from the work maternity professionals carry out within their sphere of practice. However, there are limited opportunities for caring for women and families who are experiencing bereavement. As a consequence, it is often an experienced maternity care provider who is ascribed the role of caring for women in this situation, which makes it problematical for those who are inexperienced to gain familiarity in dealing with this complex situation.

Mander (2006) reports that, for three main reasons, midwives and allied health professional's encounter difficulties in coping with perinatal death:

1. Western societies, due to sophisticated technology, more often than not find death of a baby unexpected and therefore shocking. It is often easier to accept a death of an older person.
2. Midwives may feel that they have let the mother and her family down. In other words, that the profession has not succeeded in helping a mother give birth to a healthy baby. Since childbirth is considered a routine part of life, when a

Activity 19

Contemplate how you now feel about providing care to a bereaved woman, partner and family. Consider:

- what you would say to the bereaved woman, partner and family
- what constitutes a suitable environment for a bereaved woman and family within the hospital setting
- how you may be affected by a childbearing woman's loss.

....

....

....

....

....

....

....

....

....

....

....

....

mother herself has died, the midwife may feel she has failed to accomplish the usual anticipated successful outcome.

3. Some health and social care professionals have little experience of caring for people who have encountered bereavement. Also, they may have had minimal encounters with death in their personal lives. As a result, they may feel ill-equipped to provide appropriate emotional support.

These three factors may, for some, make dealing with a bereaved woman and family a particularly stressful aspect of work. It is therefore essential that care providers recognise colleagues who require additional support in handling a bereaved woman and family. It is also the responsibility of each professional to recognise their own limitations. Care providers should learn to recognise when they are out of their depth and seek support of an experienced colleague in situations they find difficult to manage. For example, it is important to recognise when self or others have had a difficult personal experience, such as a ruptured ectopic pregnancy or traumatic birth, which may make care provision more challenging for that care provider to deal with. It is important that professionals work as a team to recognise and discuss each other's limitations and aptitudes when allocating workload.

A wealth of research has been carried out, which, in particular, examines stress experience of staff during the processes of delivering bereavement care. Peer support has been found to be one variable that affects the midwives' experience of delivering bereavement care (Kirkham, 1999; Mander, 1999; Stapleton *et al.*, 1998). So how does a leader recognise when a member of the multidisciplinary team has been affected adversely by a traumatic event or the death of a baby or mother? Stress may initially manifest itself in the form of an increase in sickness absence, or through a rise in errors in the workplace. If stress continues, a syndrome named 'burnout' may develop (Hillhouse and Adler, 1997). Such responses make recognition of stress in consequence to a death or adverse event an important concept. Team leaders must be vigilant to recognise when a member of staff is not coping well with a bereavement situation.

Within the midwifery profession there are two key players who should be mindful when a colleague is struggling with coping with a woman and family who have experienced bereavement. Firstly, the senior midwife on duty at the time of the bereavement incident, and secondly, the relevant supervisor of midwives. Specifically, when a midwife has voluntarily withdrawn from care provision, or has been removed through recognition of stress symptoms by peers. At all times, the intention should be to provide support and debriefing to that midwife and recognise training and educational needs. The goal must never be punitive.

7.1 RECOGNISING STRESS

Activity 20

Define the term 'stress':

....

....

....

....

WHAT IS STRESS?

Stress is a physical, cognitive and behavioural response to a real or imagined situation that is perceived to be threatening to our personal wellbeing.

Physiology of stress

Sympathetic response ('flight/fight' reaction)
↓
Adrenaline causes vasodilatation to muscles, heart rate ↑, respirations ↑
↓
ACTH mobilises energy
↓
If persists symptoms produced

Both physical exercise and stress are associated with sympathetic activation. In the case of exercise, free fatty acids are utilised as an energy source and are thus cleared from the circulation. If free fatty acids are not removed, as occurs when a driver is stressed by being stuck in city traffic, they can, after chemical conversion, deposit plaques of fatty material on the walls of the arteries to form atherosclerosis (Toates, 1992).

Cognitive effects of stress

Negative thoughts
Inability to make decisions
Hypersensitivity to criticism
Decreased concentration
Forgetfulness

Activity 21

Write down an episode where you felt really stressed. Recall some of
the thoughts you had:

....

....

....

....

Physical effects of stress

Palpitations
Sweating
Redness
Nausea
Urgency to go to the bathroom
Goosebumps

Activity 22

In the episode you recalled in Activity 20, recall some of the physical
symptoms you experienced:

....

....

....

....

Behavioural effects of stress

Trembling
Accident prone
Emotional outbursts
Over/under eating
Drinking
Smoking
Impulsive behaviour
Impaired speech
Nervous laughter
Restlessness

Activity 23

In the episode you recalled in Activity 20, recall some effects on your behaviour:

....

....

....

....

BEREAVEMENT AS A CAUSE OF STRESS

Causes of stress or stressors fall into two categories labelled:

1   external stressors
2   internal stressors.

EXTERNAL STRESSORS

External stressors consist of physical stimuli within the person's environment, e.g. uncomfortable hot or cold temperatures. Alternatively, the external stimuli may be an abusive colleague or being given too much work to cope with within a given time period.

INTERNAL STRESSORS

Internal stressors consist of stimuli contained within the person's body, e.g. infection, inflammation, lack of sleep, hunger or thirst. Alternatively, the internal stimuli may be psychological in origin, e.g. experiencing worrying thoughts, unpleasant dreams or anxiety. Stressors are also described as short-term (acute) or long-term (chronic):

Short-term *'acute' stress* is a reaction to an immediate threat. This is also known as the *fight or flight* response. When stress results from a stimulus, the primitive part of the brain produces chemicals that prepare the body to deal with potentially harmful stressors. The purpose is to prepare the person to run away (*flight*) or defend themselves (*fight*) from, e.g. noise, overcrowding, danger, bullying or harassment, or even an imagined or recalled threatening experience. When the threat subsides the body returns to normality, which is called the *relaxation response*. The relaxation response varies among people, with different individuals recovering from acute stress at different rates.

Long-term *'chronic' stressors* are pressures that are continuous, which result in the urge to *fight* or *flight* being suppressed. Chronic stress has effects on health and performance. It has been proven beyond doubt to make people ill, and evidence is increasing as to the number of ailments and diseases caused by stress. Stress is now known to contribute to heart disease, to cause hypertension and to impair the immune system. Stress is also linked to strokes, IBS (irritable bowel syndrome), ulcers, diabetes, muscle and joint pain, miscarriage during pregnancy, allergies, alopecia and even premature tooth loss. Stress significantly reduces brain functions, such as memory, concentration and learning, all of which are central to effective performance at work. Examples of chronic stressors include ongoing pressurised work, ongoing relationship problems, isolation and persistent financial worries.

The working environment is capable of producing both acute and chronic stressors. A childbearing woman experiencing bereavement can be one stimulus that produces a stress reaction in the midwife.

OTHER TYPICAL CAUSES OF STRESS AT WORK

- Bullying or harassment, by anyone, not necessarily a person's manager
- Feeling powerless and uninvolved in determining one's own responsibilities
- Continuous unreasonable performance demands
- Lack of effective communication and conflict resolution
- Lack of job security
- Long working hours
- Excessive time away from home and family
- Office politics and conflict among staff
- A feeling that one's reward is not commensurate with one's responsibility.

INFLUENCING THE EFFECTS OF STRESS AND STRESS SUSCEPTIBILITY

A person's susceptibility to stress can be affected by any or all of the above factors in combination. Also, everyone has different tolerance levels in relation to individual stressors. Consequently, stress susceptibility is not fixed, with each person's stress tolerance changing across time. Several factors can influence a person's stress susceptibility. These include:

- childhood experiences, e.g. child abuse or domestic violence
- personality, with some personalities more stress-prone than others
- genetics, with some people having an inherited relaxation response. This is connected with serotonin levels. Serotonin is the brain's wellbeing chemical
- immunity abnormality, which results in the person having diseases such as arthritis or eczema

- lifestyle issues, such as eating a poor diet, lack of exercise and/or sleep
- duration and intensity of stressors.

HOW CAN WE MEASURE STRESS?
Crises such as death, divorce or bankruptcy can disrupt even the best stress-management regime. Different life crises have different impacts. In many cases, however, it may be possible to anticipate crises and prepare for them. It may also be useful to recognise the impact of crises that have occurred so one can take account of them appropriately.

Some very interesting work in this area has been done by Holmes and Rahe using the *Social Readjustment Scale*, which allocates a number of 'Life Crisis Units' (LCUs) to different events, so that people can evaluate them, and take action accordingly. While this approach is an over-simplification of complex situations, using LCUs can provide overall useful information. The aim is to total the number of LCUs that have occurred to a person in the prior two years.

LCUs and probability of illness
Score of   300   80%+
Score of   200–299   50%
Score of   150–199   33%

Event	LCU scores
Death of spouse	100
Divorce	73
Separation	65
Jail term	63
Death of close family member	63
Personal illness or injury	53
Marriage	50
Fired at work	47
Marital reconciliation	45
Retirement	45

Change in health of family member	44
Pregnancy	40
Sex difficulties	39
Gain of new family member	39
Business readjustment	38
Change in financial state	38
Death of close friend	37
Change to a different line of work	36
Change in number of arguments with spouse	35
A large mortgage or loan	30
Foreclosure of mortgage or loan	30
Change in responsibilities at work	29
Son or daughter leaving home	29
Trouble with in-laws	29
Outstanding personal achievement	28
Spouse begins or stops work	26
Begin or end of school or college	26
Change in living conditions	25
Change in personal habits	24
Trouble with boss	23
Change in work hours or conditions	20
Change in residence	20
Change in school or college	20
Change in recreation	19
Change in church activities	19
Change in social activities	18
A moderate loan or mortgage	17
Change in sleeping habits	16
Change in number of family get-togethers	15
Change in eating habits	15
Holiday	13
Christmas	12
Minor violations of law	11

When one recognises in one's self or others the danger of suffering the ill effects of life crises, they should attempt to minimise disturbance to their life. If, for example, they have experienced bereavement try to avoid additional stressors.

SIGNS OF STRESS: STRESS TEST

At a clinical level, stress in individuals can be assessed scientifically by measuring the levels of two hormones produced by the adrenal glands – cortisol and DHEA (De Hydro Epi Androsterone). However, ordinarily, midwives and managers do not have ready access to such methods. They must therefore rely on other signs to identify when a person is stressed. Some of these are not exclusively due to stress, nor are they certain proof of stress. They are merely indicators to prompt investigation as to whether stress is present. You can use this list of ten key stress indicators as a simple initial stress test. Tick the factors applicable:

- sleep difficulties
- loss of appetite
- poor concentration or poor memory retention
- performance dip
- uncharacteristic errors or missed deadlines
- anger or tantrums
- violent or antisocial behaviour
- emotional outbursts
- alcohol or drug abuse
- nervous habits.

Activity 24

How did you do?

LCUs and probability of illness scale:

....

....

Signs of stress: stress test:

....

....

SLEEP DEPRIVATION AND STRESS

Healthy tiredness – There is a satisfying tiredness which follows a hard day's mental activity, i.e. a hard day decorating, a strenuous round of golf or jogging in the park. Healthy tiredness is removed through sleep and relaxation.

Unhealthy tiredness – This does not result from hard work and is present in spite of a good night's sleep. It manifests itself as mental apathy, lack of physical energy, emotional flatness and absence of highs and laughter. Unhealthy tiredness will not ease with sleep.

METHODS OF STRESS MANAGEMENT AND RELIEF

When a professional within a team recognises signs of stress in his/her self or a staff member, in this case in relation to managing a woman and bereaved family, they must not ignore it. It is their duty to act. You must refer the situation to someone who is equipped to deal with it. In addition, the midwife must also look for signs of non-work related stressors or factors that may increase a colleague's susceptibility to stress, because these will make that person more vulnerable to not coping with tricky situations in the workplace.

Stress relief methods are many and various. There is no single remedy that applies to every person suffering from stress, and most solutions involve a combination of remedies. Successful stress management frequently relies on reducing stress susceptibility and removing the stressors. Here are some simple pointers for reducing stress susceptibility and stress itself, for both yourself and others.

Stress relief pointers

1. Think seriously about and talk with others to identify the cause of the stress. Knowing what you are dealing with is essential when developing appropriate stress management approaches.
2. Remove the stressed person from the situation.
3. Eat a healthy diet. Group B vitamins and magnesium are important.

4. Reduce toxin intake, tobacco and excessive alcohol intake especially, because they work against homeostasis of the body and contribute to stress susceptibility. Therefore they increase stress itself.
5. Take exercise; it burns up adrenaline and produces endorphins, which create positive feelings.
6. Share worries. Talk to colleagues. Discussion will help colleagues understand.
7. Consider relaxation therapy, e.g. yoga, meditation, self-hypnosis or massage.

Acceptance, cognisance and commitment on the part of the stressed person are essential. No one can begin to manage their stress when they are still feeling acutely stressed, as they continuously are in *fight* or *flight* mode. The identified stressful situation must be handled by someone who will not perpetuate the stressful influence by, for example, bullying the person concerned. Removing the stressor(s) or the person from the stressful situation is only part of the solution. It is also important to look at factors that affect the person's stress susceptibility. Where possible, try to improve factors that could possibly contribute to stress vulnerability. For example, improve diet and increase levels of exercise.

ANGER MANAGEMENT AND STRESS
The term 'anger management' is widely used now as if the subject stands alone. However, anger management is simply an aspect of managing stress, since anger in the workplace is a symptom of stress. Anger is often stress in denial and as such is best approached via one-to-one counselling. Training courses can convey anger management and stress reduction theory and ideas, with counselling necessary to turn theory into practice. Management of anger and the stress that causes it can only be improved if the person wants to change. This involves acceptance, cognisance and commitment. Consequently, awareness is the first requirement. Some angry people take pride in their anger and do

not want to change. Others fail to appreciate the effects on self and others. Without a commitment to change there is not a lot that a manager or employer can do to help. Anger management is only possible when the angry person accepts and commits to the need for change.

A big factor in persuading someone of the need to commit to change is to look objectively and sensitively with that person at the consequences for self and others of their anger. Often angry people are in denial, and removing this denial is essential. Helping angry people realise that their behaviour is destructive and negative is an important first step. If the problem is a temporary tendency, then short-term acute stress may be the direct cause. One-to-one counselling may help discover the causes, followed by agreeing a plan of action to deal with the colleague. Where anger is persistent, frequent and ongoing, long-term chronic stress is more likely to be the cause. Again, counselling is required to get to the root cause. Exposing these issues can be very difficult, so sensitivity is required. The counsellor may need several sessions in order to build sufficient trust and rapport.

Where a deep and persistent upset has been caused through dealing with a childbearing woman's loss, the midwife may be willing to be referred to a suitably qualified counsellor who can help unravel their personal situation. Identifying the cause is sufficient for most people to make changes and improve. The will to change, combined with awareness of cause, often leads to resolution.

The solutions are more complex than blaming people for not being able to cope with a situation. Existing staff and new people in stress-prone roles are also likely to benefit from relaxation techniques, stress relief strategies, meditation, peace of mind and wellbeing workshops, all of which work towards increasing personal reserves necessary to deal with stressful situations. This approach, in turn, may work towards reducing absenteeism and staff loss.

PREVENTING STRESS SPECIFICALLY FROM DEALING WITH A WOMAN'S BEREAVEMENT

Prevention of undue stress can be achieved by meeting the training needs of staff involved in the care of women where there is potential for an adverse outcome. For example, during student midwife training, mentors commonly protect the student midwife from facing situations where mortality is likely. It is a mistaken belief that the student midwife should be cosseted from this kind of situation, since she can only become experienced through exposure. Once qualified, this midwife will lack the experience required to minimise stress during such situations. Ideally, the student should be exposed to bereavement situations during midwifery education, with encounters handled in a supportive way. The student should be provided with opportunities to reflect and discuss appropriate management. To promote thinking about how a bereavement incident may cause a midwife stress, consider the following activity:

Activity 25

Rebecca is a midwife who has just returned to work after having a miscarriage and she tells the ward manager that although she feels physically well, she is still upset at losing her baby. Due to staff shortage, Rebecca has been requested to help out in the early pregnancy assessment unit. How do you react to this request and why?

....

....

....

....

....

....

....

....

....

....

Maternity unit managers, lecturers and supervisors should take responsibility for continuing to provide support to colleagues while they gain experience in all areas of practice. Reducing stress can be helped by ensuring that there are adequate staffing numbers. This will allow the carer to encounter bereavement situations, firstly as an observer and subsequently taking more responsibility over time.

Encouraging continuing professional development through becoming actively involved in support groups will also provide opportunity to observe parents over a long period of time. Such opportunities facilitate staff and parents to explore ways in which difficult situations can be managed.

CONCLUSION

The objective of this chapter is to recognise where a bereavement incident has affected a peer member of staff adversely. In a completely different vein, Chapter 8 addresses the salience of professionals respecting and understanding women's spiritual and religious needs and the importance of adapting bereavement care to accommodate these where possible. Providing choice and control to women involves respecting their ideologies, attitudes and beliefs. Ascertaining women's views requires successful communication and their empowerment to have confidence to be honest.

8

Assessment and care of a bereaved woman and family's spiritual and religious needs

---

Learning objective addressed

On completion of Chapter 8 the reader should be able to:

8. Assess individual woman/partner/family's spiritual/religious beliefs and adapt bereavement care to accommodate.

Bereavement will ripple in effect to many people outside the immediate family. Extended family and friends are also likely to grieve for what has been lost. Family dynamics vary. Not all family members are close-knit, whilst others may communicate daily. Strong religious and cultural beliefs may also influence the extent and way in which each family grieves. Within each unit, friends and family will react in their own special and individual way. Consequently, professionals who come into contact with a grieving woman must adapt their support behaviour accordingly to meet each family's spiritual and religious needs.

Researchers have identified gender differences in the application of the process of grieving. Parkes (1996) and Stroebe and Schut (1999) identify hesitation and oscillation between stages as a

Activity 26

Reflect on members of the extended family who may have an essential role to play in a woman coming to terms with bereavement. Jot down some thoughts about what role these individuals may play in supporting the childbearing woman during her bereavement process.

Woman's partner:

....

....

....

Woman's brother:

....

....

....

Woman's sister:

....

....

....

Woman's father:

....

....

....

Woman's mother:

....

....

....

Woman's aunt:

....

....

....

Woman's uncle:

....

....

....

Woman's close friends:

....

....

....

component of gender differences, with a feminine passive style of grieving compared to a more active masculine style. Care must be taken by health professionals to be aware of these gender differences, but not to stereotype, since styles may differ between individuals. Recent thoughts have interpreted these styles as a logical interpretation between two distinctive coping styles (Mander, 2006).

8.1 EFFECTS OF FAMILY BEREAVEMENT ON CHILDREN

Children develop their attitudes and behaviours by observing those around them. Many families feel that it is better for children not to be too involved in the more distressing aspects of life, with the intention of protecting them from the anxieties and later inevitabilities of a death in the family. As such, these children may become puzzled by what is going on when bereavement actually occurs in the family. The child may recognise that their mother is deeply distressed, but feel incapable of comforting her. Lack of experience may lead the child to being ill-equipped to deal with grief in their adult lives.

Activity 27

Reflect on your own beliefs about discussing death with children. At what age do you think:

(a) children should be told about a person's death?
(b) children understand the irreversible truth about death?

....
....
....
....

Explore the underpinning of your thoughts on this matter:

....
....
....
....

It is rare for a child not to be faced with the reality of loss and change during their childhood. Children will usually face bereavement through the loss of a relative or even a friend. When someone close dies, adults are commonly so wound-up in their own grief that they may fail to notice that their children are also grieving. A child's grief must be handled sensitively and truthfully, and will depend on their understanding of the concept of death.

Brown (2009) proposes that children progress in their understanding of death in the subsequent manner, with understandings dependent upon the extent to which the family includes the child in discussions and upon the cultural and emotional reactions they are exposed to.

Children of 7 years and under do not understand the permanence of death. They may react adversely to the absence of a close relation who was previously involved in their day-to-day routine, but fundamentally believe that being dead means being away or asleep.

Children of 8–11 are beginning to realise that death is permanent and that it can happen to anyone. They usually expect it only to occur in older members of the family. How the child grieves will differ incalculably from overt sadness to an apparent acceptance of the event. However, the child may deny their own feelings.

Children of 12 years and above usually fully understand the finality of death. They generally wish to be involved in the arrangements for the funeral, but may turn to friends outside the family to talk about their emotions and to explore the concept of bereavement.

Telling children about a death, especially when they are toddlers, can be very difficult. The midwife's role in supporting women who ask how to 'break the news' to other children can be challenging, as she/he may not be fully cognisant of their own attitude to life and death. The person closest to the child is usually the best person to explain the situation, even though they may be in the throes of grief. The midwife can suggest that the parents relate the news in a peaceful and familiar environment. The midwife may also point out that it is important for the child to develop an understanding of what has happened in order to develop their skills for life. Using simple terminology to explain what has happened will allow the family to acknowledge the shared loss and facilitate grieving together. If the midwife is asked to be a part of this discussion, she should be open and honest and not relate the death to a non-factual circumstance. For example, she should not explain that the dead person is 'asleep' since this portrays that the death is reversible.

8.2 RELIGIOUS AND CULTURAL BELIEFS

Beliefs are formed in childhood and adopted from parents and guardians who influence the child. Attitudes are a way of being set towards or against particular pattern of beliefs. Allport (1935) states that attitude is a mental and neural state of readiness. This attitude is organised through experience that exerts a directive or dynamic influence upon the individual's response to all objects and situations with which it is related. In this instance we are talking about bereavement. Allport emphasises four basic aspects of attitudes:

1. Attitudes are internal (within neural networks).
2. Attitudes are learned (organised through experience).
3. Attitudes are response-related (a stimulus triggers the neural network).
4. Object-orientated (towards a stimuli, e.g. religious practice and belief).

As stated in point 1, attitudes are internal, i.e. stored in neural networks within the brain. These neural networks have been (2) reorganised through past experience in relation to the object of concern. In this case a past bereavement and its associated rituals are seen to be appropriate responses. Attitude stances in relation to how to react to a loss are learned through socialisation. We acquire most beliefs about a particular topic quite directly. We hear or read a fact or opinion, or other people reinforce our statements by expressing a particular attitude (Carlson, 1993). For example, a family member may say to a child, 'pull yourself together and stop crying'. Conversely, parents may applaud their child's tears in relation to the bereavement. Children in particular form attitudes through imitating or modelling the behaviour of people who play an important role in their lives. Children usually repeat opinions expressed by their parents. The tendency to identify with the family unit, and later with peer groups, provides a strong incentive to adopt group attitudes (Carlson, 1993).

Scobie (1978) explains that once an attitude has been established it develops some resistance to change. This has profound implications for the midwife who is supporting a grieving woman and her family, as they may not accept some of the behaviours that are suggested may help. For example, the concept of touching their dead infant post-delivery may not be acceptable to them.

Attitudes are underpinned by ideologies and expressed as opinions. Ideologies underpin attitudes and orientate characteristic ways of thinking about the bereavement and how to behave. In other words, ideologies provide an underlying template that directs thoughts:

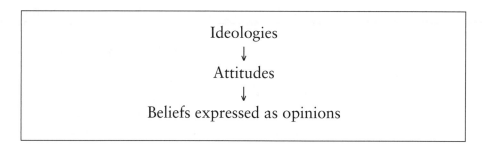

Aspects of personality also influence how a person responds to the situation. For example, an individual with the underlying ideological dimension of conservatism may manifest with personality characteristics, such as stimulus aversion and risk avoidance. These characteristic ways of thinking will be revealed through opinions expressed in conversation. Opinions are often withheld if social pressure is exerted. This may make it difficult for a health or social care professional to ascertain the woman's true opinion about what it is that has been suggested.

Care providers should provide choice and control to women in their care. This means that they must respect a woman's ideologies, attitudes and opinions (beliefs). Ascertaining women's views requires successful communication and the empowerment of women to have the confidence to be honest about expressing their opinions. Robertson (1997) provided eight key points that facilitate empowerment of women to make decisions and express views:

1. Ensure accurate information is provided.
2. The specific points where choice is available are detailed and defined.
3. The advantages and disadvantages of the various options are outlined.
4. Enough time is given for consideration of the physical and psychological implications of each choice.
5. There is information included about potential risks, flowing from specific decisions, presented in a sensitive, non-threatening manner.
6. Crisis decisions are delegated to the healthcare professionals.
7. Emotional support is available, regardless of the decision made.
8. Evaluation is made to ensure that information is understood.

Katbamna (2000) identifies that there is wide variation in the ways different cultures display grief and the mourning rituals that accompany bereavement. Veneration of the dead is based on the belief that the deceased have continued existence and possess the ability to influence the fortune of the living. Many communities venerate their ancestors. For example, the Catholic Church venerates the dead through saints, as intercessors with God. In contrast, within some eastern cultures the goal of veneration is to ensure the ancestors' continued wellbeing and positive disposition towards the living, which often involves asking for special favours or assistance. The purpose of veneration is underpinned by belief in an afterlife and survival of the deceased's personal identity beyond death. Cross-culturally, these beliefs are far from uniform. In some cultures people believe that their ancestors need to be provided for by their descendants. Others do not believe that the ancestors are even aware of what their descendants do for them. Instead, an expression of filial piety is what is important. The act of veneration is a way to respect, honour and care for ancestors in their afterlives, and seek guidance for their living descendants. For example, this may be by maintaining the graves of parents or other ancestors and leaving flowers to honour and remember them. In addition, midwives may be familiar with the wailing and stark displays of grief shown by some ethnic groups, with some finding it difficult to relate to these demonstrations of raw emotions. Within cultural groups, however, there can also be wide variations in emotions displayed between individuals in relation to death.

Activity 28

Ancestor veneration is practised by the Chinese and other Buddhist and Confucian-influenced societies. Take a look on the internet and identify some of the cultural practices that help members of these societies cope with their bereavement.

Examples:

1. ....
....
....

2. ....
....
....

3. ....
....
....

Schott and Henley (1996) observe that some people with strong religious faith gain strength and comfort from their spiritual and religious belief systems. Others find it difficult to retain their faith and blame God for allowing this shocking loss to happen to them.

The amount of support gained through religious and cultural beliefs may vary greatly. What is found to be acceptable may be profoundly influenced by the attitude of community members and religious leaders. For example, the characteristics of the ceremony carried out to mourn the death of the infant. Whatever processes are involved, the midwife must allow the family to express grief as they see appropriate.

It would be useful for caring professionals to have some understanding of different religious and cultural beliefs about death and bereavement. Mander (2006) states that sometimes maternity care providers encounter difficulties accepting differing attitudes to loss by women from cultures other than their own. Mander goes on to question whether care providers are able to work through these feelings in order to support women during the grieving process. Professionals must work to overcome their intolerances. Providing support and time to listen are essential components of care provision.

Activity 29

Reflect on the different cultural groups that you have encountered during your professional practice.

What have you observed about some women's particular belief systems and their reactions to particular events?

....

....

....

....

....

....

....

8.3 THE ROLE OF RITUALS

Rituals are an important way of expressing grief and it is appropriate that parents be encouraged to plan the funeral and burial within their own cultural and belief system. Maternity care providers must be respectful of individual cultural backgrounds and ensure that parental wishes are facilitated. Families must be asked about their needs and every effort made to embrace their requested cultural and religious rituals. In order to facilitate another's grief process effectively, professionals require to be at ease with the concept of their own death. This requires that they consider what they would like to happen to them when they die.

Activity 30

Consider other structured belief systems. Find out what rituals are common practices at funerals in the following three religions:

Judaism

....

....

....

....

....

Buddhism

....

....

....

....

....

Islam

....

....

....

....

....

8.4 ENCOURAGING MEMORIES

As mentioned in Chapter 2, protocols can help shape the bereavement care that is provided within the maternity unit. An important part of following a protocol is to be flexible and accommodate parents' cultural and spiritual beliefs. As part of these protocols, midwives are required to help parents gather meaningful memories of their infant, which is designed to help them grieve appropriately and adapt to their loss:

- Gather photographs, hand or foot prints, ultrasound photograph, baby's name card.
- Take a lock of hair.
- Facilitate parents in spending time with their deceased baby.
- Support parents when viewing and holding their deceased baby.
- Use appropriate grief symbols, such as angels, candles and flowers.

These treasured items and symbols can help parents construct the infant's social identity and promote creation of constructive and concrete memories.

Conclusion

Well done for completing this work book. What has been learned will make you better equipped to cope with women and families who have experienced loss or death within the childbearing remit. This workbook may also allow you to address personal issues. The authors acknowledge that bereavement and loss are emotive subjects and the completion of this workbook may not have been an easy experience. Some time may need to be taken to reflect upon the issues raised that were particularly meaningful and perhaps difficult or painful.

Palliative care is composed of three components: pain and comfort management; assistance with end-of-life decision-making; and bereavement support. Within this delivery, maternity care providers must acknowledge their own grief for the death of an infant in their care and work to support the bereaved before, during and after this devastating experience. Grief is a journey, and by travelling the road with the woman and her family, professional carers can help validate the meaning of life. It is their charge to remain open so that they may give without breaking. During the process, it is important that maternity care providers recognise the philosophical significance of each childbearing woman's journey.

References

Abortion Act (1967) in Mason, J.K. and Laurie, G.T. (2005) *Mason and McCall Smith's Law and Medical Ethics*, 7th edn. Oxford: Oxford University Press.

American Psychiatric Association (2000) *Diagnostic and Statistical Manual of Mental Disorders*, 4th edn. *Text Revision (DSM-IV-TR)*. Washington, DC: APA.

Allport, G. (1935) 'Attitudes', in Murchison, C. (4th edn) (1985) *A Handbook of Social Psychology*. Worcester, MA: Clark University Press.

ARC (Antenatal Results and Choices) (2012) Available at: http://www.arc-uk.org/ (accessed 1 March 2012).

Badenhorst, W., Riches, S., Turton, P. and Hughes, P. (2006) 'The psychological effects of stillbirth and neonatal death on fathers: systematic review'. *Journal of Psychosomatic Obstetrics and Gynaecology*, 27(4): 245–56.

Barr, P. and Cacciatore, J. (2008) 'Personal fear of death and grief in bereaved mothers'. *Death Studies*, 32: 445–60.

Bartellas, E. and Van Aerde, J. (2003) 'Bereavement support for women and their families after stillbirth'. *Journal of Obsterics and Gynaecology Canada*, 25(2): 131–8.

Billson, A. and Tyrrell, J. (2003) 'How to break bad news'. *Current Paediatrics*, 13: 284–7.

Blackburn, C. and Copley, R. (1989) 'One precious moment: what you can offer when a newborn infant dies'. *Nursing*, 19: 52–4.

Bonanno, G. A. (2009) *The Other Side of Sadness: What the New Science of Bereavement Tells Us About Life After Loss*. New York: Basic Books.

Borg, J. (2010) *Body Language: 7 Easy Lessons to Master the Silent Language*. New Jersey: FT Press.

Bourne, P. (1968) 'The psychological effects of stillbirth on women and their doctors'. *Journal of the Royal College of General Practitioners*, 16: 103–12.

Bowlby, J. (1961) 'Processes of mourning'. *International Journal of Psychoanalysis*, 44(317).

Bowlby, J. (1981) *Attachment and Loss*, Vol. 3, 1st edn. New York, Basic Books.

Bowlby, J. (1990) *The Making and Breaking of Affectionate Bonds*. London: Routledge.

Brier, N. (2008) 'Grief following miscarriage: a comprehensive review of the literature'. *Journal of Women's Health*, 17(3): 451–64.

Brost, L. and Kenney, J. (1992) 'Pregnancy after perinatal loss: parental reactions and nursing interventions'. *Journal of Obstetric Gynecologic and Neonatal Nursing*, 21: 457–63.

Brown, E. (2009) 'Helping bereaved children and young people'. *British Journal of School Nursing*, 4(2): 69–73.

Brown, Y. (1993) 'Perinatal loss: a framework for good practice'. *Health Care for Women International*, 14: 469–79.

Büchi, S., Mörgeli, H., Schynder, U., Jenewin, J., Glaser, A., Fauchère, J. C., Bucher, H. and Sensky, T. (2008) 'Shared or discordant grief in couples 2–6 years after the death of their premature baby: effects on suffering and posttraumatic growth'. *Psychosomatics*, 50(2): 123–30.

Caelli, K., Downie, J. and Letendre, A. (2002) 'Parent's experiences of midwife-managed care following the loss of a baby in a previous pregnancy'. *Journal of Advanced Nursing*, 39(2): 127–36.

Calhoun, B., Napolitano, P., Terry, M., Bussey, C. and Hoeldtke, N. (2003) 'Perinatal hospice: comprehensive care for the family of the fetus with a lethal condition'. *Journal of Reproductive Medicine*, 48(5): 343–8.

Capitulo, K. (2005) 'Evidence for healing interventions with perinatal bereavement'. *American Journal of Maternal Child Nursing*, 30(6): 389–96.

Carlson, N. (1993) *Psychology: The Science of Behaviour*. London: Allyn and Bacon, p. 583.

Centre for Maternal and Child Enquiries (CMACE) (2011) 'Saving mother's lives: reviewing maternal deaths to make motherhood safer: 2006–2008'. The Eighth Report on Confidential Enquiries into Maternal Deaths in the United Kingdom. *BJOG, An International Journal of Obstetrics & Gynaecology*, 118(suppl. 1): 1–223.

Condon, J. (2010) 'Women's mental health: a wish-list for the DSM V'. *Archives* of *Women's Mental Health*, 13: 5–10.

Côté-Arsenault, D. and Morrison-Beedy, D. (2001) 'Support groups helping women through pregnancies after loss'. *Western Journal of Nursing Research*, 26(6): 650–70.

Davies, R. (2004) 'New understandings of parental grief: literature review'. *Journal of Advanced Nursing*, 46(5): 506–13.

DeBackere, K., Hill, P. and Kavanagh, K. (2008) 'The parental experience of pregnancy after perinatal loss'. *Journal of Obstetric, Gynecologic & Neonatal Nursing*, 37(5): 525–37.

Engel, G.C. (1961) 'Is grief a disease? A challenge for medical research'. *Psychosomatic Medicine*, 23: 18–22.

Engelhard, I., van den Hout, M. and Arntz, A. (2001) 'Posttraumatic stress disorder after pregnancy loss'. *General Hospital Psychiatry*, 21: 62–6.

Engler, A.J., Cusson, R.M. and Brockett, R.T. (2004) 'Neonatal staff and advanced practice nurses' perceptions of bereavement/end-of-life care of families of critically ill and /or dying infants'. *American Journal of Critical Care*, 13: 489–98.

Engler A.J. and Lasker, J.N. (2000) 'Predictors of maternal grief in the year after a newborn death". *Illness, Crisis and Loss*, 8: 227–43.

Enkin, M., Keirse, M., Renfrew, M. and Neilson, J. (1995) *A Guide to Effective Care in Pregnancy and Childbirth*, 2nd edn. Oxford: Oxford University Press.

Gardner, J. M. (1999) 'Perinatal death: uncovering the needs of midwives and nurses and exploring helpful interventions in the United States, England, and Japan'. *Journal of Transcultural Nursing*, 10: 120–30.

Gensch, B. K. and Midland, D. (2000) 'When a baby dies: a standard of care'. *Illness, Crisis and Loss*, 8: 286–95.

Government Statistical Service (2006) *Statistical Bulletin Abortion Statistics, England and Wales: 2005*. Available at: www.dh.gov.uk/assetRoot/04/13/68/59/04136859.pdf (accessed on 19 August 2012).

Hertz, R. ([1907] 1960) *Death and the Right Hand*. Aberdeen: Cohen and West.

Hillhouse, J.J. and Adler C.M. (1997) 'Investigating stress effect patterns in hospital staff nurses: results of a cluster analysis'. *Social Science and Medicine,* 45(12): 1781–8.

Hollins Martin, C. J. (2008) 'Birth planning for midwives and mothers'. *British Journal of Midwifery,* 16(9): 583–7.

Hughes, P., Turton, P., Hopper, E. and Evans, C. (2002) 'Assessment of guidelines for good practice in psychosocial care of mothers after stillbirth: a cohort study'. *Lancet*, 360: 114–18.

Jones, A. (1989) 'Managing the invisible grief'. *Senior Nurse*, 9(5): 26–7.

Katbamna, S. (2000) *Race and Childbirth*. Buckingham: Open University Press.

Kavanaugh, K., Trier, D. and Korzec, M. (2004) 'Social support following perinatal loss'. *Journal of Family Nursing*, 10: 70–92.

Kelly, E. (2007) *Marking Short Lives: Constructing and Sharing Rituals following Pregnancy Loss*. Oxford: Peter Lang.

Kendler, K., Myers, J. and Zisook, S. (2008) 'Does bereavement-related major depression differ from major depression associated with other stressful life events?' *American Journal of Psychiatry*, 165(11): 1449–55.

Kennel, J.H. and Klaus, M.H. (1970) 'The mourning response of parents to death of a newborn infant'. *New England Journal of Medicine*, 283: 344–9.

Kennel, J.H. and Traause, M.A. (1978) 'Helping parents cope with perinatal death'. *Contemporary OB/GYN*, 12: 53–68.

Kirkham, M. (1999) 'The culture of midwifery in the National Health Service in England'. *Journal of Advanced Nursing*, 30(3): 732–9.

Kirkley-Best, E. and Kellner, K.R. (1982) 'Forgotten grief: a review of the literature on the psychology of stillbirth'. *American Journal of Orthopsychiatry*, 52: 420–9.

Klass, D. (1996) 'The deceased child in the psychic and social worlds of bereaved parents during resolution of grief' in Klass, D., Silvermann, P. and Nickman, S. (eds) (1999) *Continuing Bonds: New Understandings of Grief*. London: Taylor and Francis.

Klass, D., Silverman, P. and Nickman, S. (1996) *Continuing Bonds: New Understandings of Grief*. Washington, DC: Taylor and Francis.

Kroth, J., Garcia, M., Hallgren, M., LeGrue, E., Ross, M. and Scalise, J. (2004) 'Perinatal loss, trauma and dream reports'. *Psychological Reports*, 94(31): 877–82.

Kübler-Ross, E. (1969) *On Death and Dying*. New York: Macmillan.

Kübler-Ross, E. and Kessler, D. (2005) *On Grief and Grieving: Finding the Meaning of Grief through the Five Stages of Loss*. New York: Scribner.

LaRoche, C., Lalinec-Michaud, M., Engelsmann, F., Fuller, N., Copp, M. and McQuade-Soldatos, L. (1984) 'Grief reactions to perinatal death'. *Canadian Journal of Psychiatry*, 29: 14–19.

Lasker, J.N. and Toedter, L.J. (1991) 'Acute versus chronic grief: the case of pregnancy loss'. *American Journal of Orthopsychiatry*, 61(4): 510–22.

Lasker, J.N. and Toedter, L.J. (2000) 'Predicting outcomes after pregnancy loss: results from studies using the perinatal grief scale'. *Illness, Crisis and Loss*, 8(4): 350–72.

Leon, I.G. (1992) 'Perinatal loss: a critique of current hospital practices'. *Clinical Pediatrics*, 31: 366–74.

Lewis, G. (2004) Confidential Enquiry into Maternal and Child Health (CEMACH) *Why Mother's Die: Sixth Report on Confidential Enquiries into Maternal Deaths in the United Kingdom 2000–2002*. London: RCOG Press.

Lewis, G. (2007) Confidential Enquiry into Maternal and Child Health (CEMACH) *Why Mother's Die: Seventh Report on Confidential Enquiries into Saving Mothers Lives: Reviewing Maternal Deaths to Make Motherhood Safer 2003–2005*. London: RCOG Press.

Lin, S.X. and Lasker, J.N. (1996) 'Patterns of grief reaction after pregnancy loss'. *American Journal of Orthopsychiatry*, 66: 262–71.

Lindemann, E. (1944) 'Symptomatology and management of acute grief'. *American Journal of Psychiatry*, 101: 141–9.

Lok, I. and Neugebauer, R. (2007) 'Psychological morbidity following miscarriage'. *Best Practice and Research Clinical Obstetrics and Gynaecology*, 21(2): 229–47.

McHaffie, H. (2001) *Crucial Decisions at the Beginning of Life*. Abingdon: Radcliffe Medical Press.

Mander, R. (1999) 'The death of a mother: a proposed research project'. *RCM Midwives' Journal*, 2(1): 24–5.

Mander, R. (2006) *Loss and Bereavement in Childbearing*, 2nd edn. London: Routledge.

Mehta, P. (2008) 'Communication skills – breaking bad news'. *Pediatrics in Practice*, 45: 839–41.

Midwifery 2020 UK Programme (2010) *Midwifery 2020: Delivering Expectations*. Edinburgh: Midwifery 2020 UK Programme.

NES (NHS Education for Scotland) (2006) *A Curricular Framework for Perinatal Mental Health*. Edinburgh: NES.

Ngan Kee, W.D. (2005) 'Confidential enquiries into maternal deaths: 50 years of closing the loop'. *British Journal of Anaesthesia*, 94(4): 413–16.

Ngo-Metzer, Q. (2009) 'Breaking bad news over the phone'. *American Family Physician*, 80(5): 521–22.

NICE (National Institute for Health and Clinical Excellence) (2007) *Antenatal and Postnatal Mental Health: Clinical Management and Service Guidance*. London: NICE.

Nicol, M.T., Tompkins, J.R., Campbell, N.A. and Syme, G.J. (1986) 'Maternal grieving response after perinatal death'. *Medical Journal Australia*, 144: 287–9.

NMC (Nursing and Midwifery Council) (2010) *Midwives' Rules and Standards*. London: NMC.

NMSF (National Maternity Support Foundation) (2009) *Who Care When You Lose a Baby: A Comprehensive Study into Bereavement Midwife Care across NHS Trusts*. National Maternity Support Foundation (NMSF).

O'Connor, M.F., Irwin, M.R. and Wellisch, D.K. (2009) 'When grief heats up: pro-inflammatory cytokines predict regional brain activation'. *Neuroimage*, 47: 891–6.

O'Lunaigh, P. and Carlson, C. (2005) *Midwifery and Public Health*. Edinburgh: Elsevier.

Parkes, C.M. (1996) *Bereavement: Studies of Grief in Adult Life*, 3rd edn. London: Tavistock.

Pavlish, C. (2005) 'Action responses in Congolese refugee women'. *Journal of Nursing Scholarship*, 37(1): 10–17.

Price, S. (2007) *Mental Health in Pregnancy and Childbirth*. Philadelphia, PA: Churchill Livingstone.

Radestad, I., Steineck, G., Nordin, C. and Sjogren, B. (1996) 'Psychological complications after stillbirth: influence of memories and immediate management: population based study'. *British Medical Journal*, 312: 1505.

Raynor, M. and England, C. (2010) *Psychology for Midwives*. Glasgow: McGraw Hill.

Reiger, K.M. and Lane, K.L. (2009) 'Working together: collaboration between midwives and doctors in public hospitals'. *Australian Health Review*, 33(2): 315–24.

Reena, K. (2005) *Body Language in Patient Counselling. AECS Illumination*, 5(1): 25–7.

Robertson, A. (1997) *Empowering Women*. Camperdown: Ace Graphics, p. 64.

Robinson, M., Baker, L. and Nackerud, L. (1999) 'The relationship between attachment theory and perinatal loss'. *Death Studies*, 23: 257–70.

Romm, J. (2002) 'Breaking bad news in obstetrics and gynaecology: educational conference for resident physicians'. *Archives of Women's Mental Health*, 5: 177–9.

Rowe, J., Clyman, R., Green, C., Mikkelson, C., Haight, J. and Ataide, L. (1978) 'Follow-up of families who experience a perinatal death'. *Pediatrics*, 62: 166–70.

Rowa-Dewar, N. (2002) 'Do interventions make a difference to bereaved parents? A systematic review of controlled studies'. *International Journal of Palliative Nursing*, 8: 452–7.

Royal College of Obstetricians and Gynaecologists (RCOG) (2001a) 'Further issues relating to late abortion, fetal viability and registration of births and deaths'. Available at: www.rcog.org.uk/index.asp?PageID_549 (accessed on 18 August 2012).

Säflund, K., Sjögren, B. and Wredling, R. (2004) 'The role of caregivers after a stillbirth: views and experiences of parents'. *Birth*, 31, 132–7.

SANDS (Stillbirth and Neonatal Death Society) (2009) *Miscarriage, Stillbirth and Neonatal Death*. London: SANDS.

Schott, J. and Henley, A. (1996) *Culture, Religion and Childbearing in a Multiracial Society*. Oxford: Butterworth Heinemann.

Scobie, G. (1978) 'Teaching in social attitude areas'. *Association of Educational Psychologists*, 4(8): 13–15.

Scottish Government (2011) *Shaping Bereavement Care – A Framework for Action*. Available from: www.sehd.scot.nhs.uk/mels/CEL2011_09.pdf (accessed 28 July 2011).

Séjourné, N., Callahan, S. and Chabrol, H. (2010) 'Support following miscarriage: what women want'. *Journal of Reproductive and Infant Psychology*, 28(4): 403–11.

Shane, M. (1992) *Enduring, Sharing, Loving*. London: Darton, Longman and Todd.

Stack, C.G. (2003) 'Bereavement in paediatric intensive care'. *Paediatric Anaesthesia*, 13: 651–4.

Stapleton, H., Duerden, J. and Kirkham, M. (1998) *Evaluation of the Impact of the Supervision of Midwives on Professional Practice and the Quality of Midwifery Care*. London: University of Sheffield and ENB for Nursing, Midwifery and Health Visiting.

Statham, H., Solomou, W. and Green, J.M. (2001) 'Care in hospital for parents who terminated their pregnancy', in *When a Baby has an Abnormality: A Study of Parents' Experiences* (Chapter 6). Cambridge: Centre for Family Research, University of Cambridge.

Statham, H. (2002) 'Prenatal diagnosis of fetal abnormality: the decision to terminate the pregnancy and the psychological consequences'. *Fetal Maternity Medical Review*, 13: 213–47.

Stroebe, M. and Schut, H. (1999) 'The dual process model of coping with bereavement: rational and description'. *Death Studies*, 23(3): 197–224.

Surkan, P., Radestad, I., Cnattingius, S., Steineck, G. and Dickman, P. (2008) 'Events after stillbirth in relation to maternal depressive symptoms: a brief report'. *Birth*. 35(2): 153–7.

Taft, P. (2009) 'Breaking bad news'. *Nursing Standard*, 24(10): 59.

Toates, F. (1992) *Biology Brain and Behaviour: Control of Behaviour*. Milton Keynes: Open University.

Toedter, L.J., Lasker, J.N. and Alhadeff, J.M. (1988) 'The perinatal grief scale: development and initial validation'. *American Journal of Orthopsychiatry*, 58: 435–49.

Walsh, D. and Gamble, J. (2005) 'Multidisciplinary collaboration and team work misnomers for subjugation'. *Australian Midwifery*, 18(3): 7–8.

Walter, T. (1999) *On Bereavement: The Culture of Grief*. Philadelphia, PA: Open University Press.

Whitney, S., McCullough, L.B., Frugé, E., McGuire, A. and Volk, R. (2008) 'Beyond breaking bad news'. *American Cancer Society*, 113(2): 442–5.

WHO (World Health Organisation) (2010) 'International statistical classification of diseases and related health problems (10th revision) (Vol. 1): Tabular list (Vol. 2): Instruction manual'. Geneva: WHO.

WHO (World Health Organisation) (2012) 'WHO/UNICEF/UNFPA/ The World Bank: trends in maternal mortality: 1990 to 2010'. Geneva: WHO, UNICEF, UNFPA and The World Bank estimates.

Williams, C., Munson, D., Zupanic, J. and Kirpalani, H. (2008) 'Supporting bereaved parents: practical steps in providing compassionate perinatal and neonatal end-of-life care: A North American perspective'. *Fetal and Neonatal Medicine*, 13: 335–40.

Worden, J.W. (1983) *Grief Counselling and Grief Therapy*, 1st edn. London: Tavistock.

Worden, J.W. (1991) *Grief Counselling and Grief Therapy*, 2nd edn. London: Routledge.

Yentis, S. M. (2011) 'From CEMD to CEMACH to CMACE to…? Where now for the confidential enquiries into maternal deaths?' *Anaesthesia*, 66(10): 859–60.

Zeanah, C. H. (1989) 'Adaptation following perinatal loss: a critical review'. *American Academy of Child Adolescent Psychiatry*, 28(3): 467–80.

Index